THE DIET PILL GUIDE

D1236153

Also by Deborah R. Mitchell

Nature's Painkillers
Broccoli Sprouts Breakthrough
The Dictionary of Natural Healing

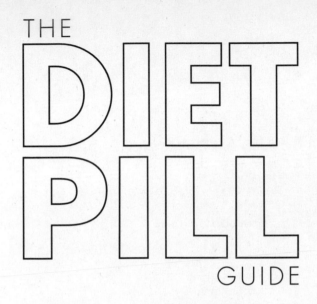

THE DIET PILL GUIDE

THE CONSUMER'S BOOK OF OVER-THE-COUNTER AND PRESCRIPTION WEIGHT-LOSS PILLS AND SUPPLEMENTS

Deborah R. Mitchell

AND

David Charles Dodson, M.D.

ST. MARTIN'S GRIFFIN ☧ NEW YORK

www.stmartins.com

ISBN 0-312-28711-9

First St. Martin's Griffin Edition: January 2002

10 9 8 7 6 5 4 3 2 1

IMPORTANT NOTE

THIS BOOK is for informational purposes only. It is not intended to take the place of medical advice from a trained medical professional. Although some of the entries contain specific precautions, warnings, or directives to consult with a physician, readers should not assume that the absence of specific warnings means that the supplement is safe under all circumstances. Readers are advised to consult a physician or other qualified health professional regarding treatment of all health matters, including weight problems, before making any major changes in diet and before taking any of the supplements or drugs reviewed in this book.

The fact that an organization or Web site is listed in this book as a potential source of information does not mean that the author or publisher endorses any of the information it may provide or recommendations it may make.

Research about weight loss and weight-loss supplements is ongoing and subject to conflicting interpretations and new information. Likewise, readers should be advised that Web sites offered as sources for further information may have changed since this was written.

CONTENTS

PREFACE

THE BAD news is that Americans are the fattest people in the world. The worse news is that a never-ending parade of diets, pills, powders, and potions often results only in weight loss for the dieter's wallet, and weight gain for the seller of the book or remedy. This book is a guide for the perplexed, a reference that finally explains in plain, simple terms what is in the various products on the market, how they work, or in many cases, how they don't work. This book can save its readers not only money, but also the pain and discomfort of side effects and the frustration of wasting hard-earned dollars on bogus products—not to mention the heartache of being let down when they don't work.

In 1998, the National Heart, Lung, and Blood Institute released the first federal guidelines for the management of obesity. This report redefined obesity and introduced the term *overweight* in terms of something called "body mass index" (BMI), which will be explained more fully in the Introduction. Prior to this report, obesity was simply medical jargon for being overweight and there was no separate overweight category.

At least 55 percent of Americans are overweight according to the new BMI calculation. This does not take into account bodybuilders. Arnold Schwarzenegger fits the category of "overweight but not obese" because he is overweight by virtue of his large muscle mass. However, the great majority of people with high BMI *do* have excess body fat. The problem of our increasing national girth has been worsening at an alarming rate and involves children as well as adults. One expert claimed that at the rate we've been going, all Americans will be over-weight by the year 2030! This is obviously absurd, but the fact that most American adults are overweight means our diets are quite bad.

One school of thought says "who cares, fat is beautiful, leave me alone." This is because no one has found *the solution*. Weight loss is so often followed by weight gain that we should just accept being overweight or obese as a fact of modern life. We should just quit telling overweight people to lose weight and making them feel bad. Although I personally feel much empathy for overweight patients, it is essentially a defeatist point of view. As a physician interested in preventive medicine, I must disagree. The problem is that being overweight is not merely a cosmetic issue. Indeed, Shakespeare warns the rotund Falstaff, "Leave gourmandizing. Know the grave doth gape for thee thrice wider than for other men." Obesity is not only a deadly disease, which shortens lifespan, it increases the risk for conditions such as arthritis, coronary heart disease, sleep apnea, diabetes, cancer, and other serious health problems. Despite the fat acceptance movement, we as a nation are, and are likely to remain, prejudiced against obese people.

As my hair gets grayer, I become more convinced that being overweight is very often connected to psychological issues. Most people with weight problems have struggled to lose for years and in the process have become quite expert in the fields of diet and exercise . . . yet their weight remains out of control. This implies a sort of mental block, an inability to apply the knowledge one has. For example, if a 150-pound person (on a 2,100-calorie-a-day diet) walked for 1 hour every day, that per-son would lose 36 pounds in a year; at 30 minutes a day, 18 pounds. Many people know this, yet how many are doing it? We are creatures of habit, and much as we might like to weigh less, often the motivation to make the lifestyle changes is not as strong as the desire to lose weight, and hence weight loss either doesn't happen or it is temporary as old habits are resumed and the weight inevitably returns.

Certainly changing habits is hard. It is perhaps even harder to change one's self-image. We all have an image of ourselves as looking the way we do. To think of ourselves as thinner people is not easy, yet that is exactly what we must do in order to succeed. Specialists in behavior modification can help in the effort to remake ourselves into thinner people: people who don't eat junk food (regularly), who exercise instead of vegging in front of the tube. Prayer and meditation can also help, and I recommend both to anyone as part of a weight-loss program, and as part of stress management and physical health in general.

Perhaps the most important advice in this book is found in the section on Liking Your Selves in the Introduction. If we really like ourselves, we will not abuse our bodies with calorific junk foods, and we'll come to realize the truth of the late, great Buckminster Fuller's observation that "God gave us legs, not roots."

In my fifteen years in clinical nutrition, I have seen many fads come and go. I would like to comment on two: one dietary, one a drug. Both of them are, in my medical opinion, dangerous. The drug is ephedra, contained in the Chinese herb ma huang. Ephedra is a potent stimulant that can raise blood pressure; its use has been associated with stroke, heart attack, and death. It is found in many weight-loss products and does promote weight loss. In my opinion, however, it is not worth the risk. Ephedra is discussed in more detail in Part II, and products containing it are clearly identified in Part III. Another Chinese herb, sida cordifolia, contains a different stimulant, synephrine. This substance is newer to the market and less information is available; however, I would view it with extreme caution as well. In the 1960s, the saying "speed kills" was popularized to dramatize the danger of using stimulants. That warning should not be forgotten.

High-protein diets keep coming back to haunt nutritionists. The latest versions are trumped up in pseudoscience suggesting that excess carbohydrates cause the body to become resistant to insulin and that this causes obesity and diabetes. The solution is to replace carbohydrates with protein. This theory is not based on scientific evidence and overlooks the fact that practically every society has always gotten most of its calories from carbohydrates.

For example, Asian diets are based on rice. If the carbohydrates-cause-obesity theory is correct, Asian cultures should be rife with obesity and diabetes, but of course they are not. The average Asian rice eater is slender. So much for the theory behind high-protein diets. These diets contradict all the advice given by good professional groups with science to back up their recommendations: groups including the American Academy of Pediatrics, the American Heart Association, the National Cancer Institute, the American Diabetes Association, and so on. The authors of protein diet books have made millions suggesting they are wiser than all these professional organizations. But their riches and their status as bestselling authors do not make them right and in my opinion, and in the opinion of any number of my colleagues in the nutrition field, the protein books are essentially nutritional fiction, and dangerous fiction at that. Dr. Atkins—to the contrary, steak and eggs are not health foods!

Good, healthy foods; exercise; prayer and meditation; sometimes formal behavior-modification therapy; sometimes weight-loss products—these are the keys to losing weight. But weight loss is not the main goal. All diets work in the short term. But unless you make a permanent change in your diet and exercise habits, you should expect the weight you lose to come back, usually with a vengeance. Therefore, it is best to make changes you are comfortable with and can maintain permanently. That is the only way to achieve permanent weight loss, which is the real goal. Indeed, it is better to stay overweight than to engage in "the rhythm method of girth control," also known as yo-yo dieting. This is the pitfall of crash diets, including high-protein diets. People can only stay on an unbalanced, unhealthy crash diet so long before they go off it, usually back to the same diet that caused the weight problem.

So if not carbohydrates, what does cause people to get fat? Wonder of wonders, it turns out to be fat. Only fat and alcohol are fattening. To lose weight, you must burn off more calories than you eat. This can be done by increasing your exercise and/ decreasing calories. There are four kinds of calories: fat, carbohydrate, protein, and alcohol. To get fat in the first place, you must eat fat or drink alcohol. This is why people in countries such as Japan and Korea, where rice is a staple and where fat consumption is low, remain slim. That the slimness of Asians is not a genetic trait is easily confirmed by walking around any U.S. Chinatown, where you will spot more overweight Asian-Americans in an hour than you will in the Far East in a week. I've tried the experiment.

I believe this book will be of great use not only to the dieting public, but to their health-care providers as well. The problem of being overweight is a great challenge, but not an impossible one. With the publication of this book, it has become easier, and perhaps more important, safer too.

—David Charles Dodson, M.D.,
Assistant Clinical Professor of Medicine,
Tufts University School of Medicine

The Skinny on Dieting and Dieting Products

"LOSE 30 Pounds in 30 Days Without Dieting!" "Eat All You Want and Lose Weight!" "Fast, Fun, and Effortless!" "Lose Weight While You Sleep!" If any of these things were true about losing weight, very few people would be ten, twenty, thirty, and more pounds above their ideal, healthy weight.

About 97 million American adults (55 percent) are overweight or obese, according to the National Heart, Lung, and Blood Institute. At any given time, 33 to 40 percent of women and 20 to 24 percent of men in the United States are on a diet. Many of these individuals are buying diet products or enrolling in weight-loss programs—to the tune of $33 billion-plus annually—to help them lose excess pounds.

When it comes to diet pills, most people make their purchases based on little or no reliable information. In desperation, they believe the ads and the come-ons. They've tried diet after diet and nothing seems to work. A product that promises it will allow you to lose weight even while you enjoy all the chocolate and potato chips you want sounds too good to be true. And it is—but tens of thousands of people buy it anyway. Perhaps you've bought it, too.

But you don't have to make that mistake again, because this book offers you well-researched information about various weight-loss products. It provides information to help you draw your own conclusions and make your own choices about which diet product is right—or wrong—for you.

The three main parts of this book provide important information about prescription, single-ingredient, and combination-ingredient diet products. Although there are hundreds of diet

2 · The Diet Pill Guide

products that fall into these categories, they essentially share a basic, common footnote: the manufacturers tell consumers (usually in tiny, barely readable type) that the product should be used along with a reduced-calorie diet and exercise to see results. A brief discussion about the elements of that common footnote—obesity, nutrition, and exercise—are in order to lay a foundation for the rest of the book.

AM I OVERWEIGHT OR OBESE?

Dr. Dodson introduced the term *BMI* (body mass index) in the Preface, which is now used by experts to define being overweight/obese. Simply put, the BMI is a calculation derived from height and weight. Using the BMI, individuals of different heights and weights can compare their degree of being overweight. Being overweight is defined as a BMI between 25 and 30, and obese is a BMI greater than 30. Previously, anyone with a BMI greater than 27 was considered obese, and there was no overweight category. You can determine your BMI by using the chart on pages 4 and 5.

There is another set of guidelines to help you determine the health risks of being overweight. C. Wayne Callaway, M.D., associate clinical professor of medicine at George Washington University in Washington, D.C., and a leading authority on obesity, prefers the waist-to-hip ratio method. The waist-to-hip ratio is calculated by dividing the number of inches around the waistline by the circumference of the hips. If your waist is 28 inches and your hips are 40 inches, for example, your ratio would be 0.70 (28 divided by 40). Women with a ratio of 0.8 or higher and men with a ratio of 0.95 or greater are at high risk of weight-related health problems. An easier variation, popular with nutritionists, simply looks at waist measurement: a woman whose waist is more than 36 inches or a man whose waist is more than 40 inches is at increased risk for medical problems associated with weight and should try to lose some.

HEALTH RISKS OF OVERWEIGHT/OBESITY

You've heard the warnings: being overweight contributes to serious health risks, such as heart disease, diabetes, and cancer—three of the most life-threatening medical conditions. But many other medical problems are also related to being overweight. These include high cholesterol, high blood pressure (hypertension), kidney disease, arthritis, gout, varicose veins, gallbladder disease, liver disease, menstrual problems, stroke, and infertility. If you are obese, how serious are these problems? Compared with normal-weight individuals:

- You have 2 times the risk of developing high blood pressure.
- You have an increased risk of developing colon cancer, breast cancer, and cancer of the uterus and gall bladder.
- Your chances of developing adult-onset diabetes are 3.8 times greater.
- You have a 2.1 times greater risk of getting hypercholesterolemia (high cholesterol).
- You are likely to develop arthritis at an earlier age and to have a more debilitating form (because of the stress on your joints).
- You are more likely to have menstrual problems (heavy or painful periods) and you have a greater chance of fertility problems.
- You are more likely to experience sleep apnea (cessation of respiration while asleep) and varicose veins.

Recent studies show that people who are 20 percent or more overweight can experience significant health benefits when they lose 10 to 20 pounds, including a reduction in cholesterol levels and blood pressure. Losing weight can even lengthen your life: life expectancy of people who are overweight is lower than that of normal-weight individuals. Besides health issues, obesity has a negative effect on quality of life, including low self-esteem, depression, social prejudice, and job discrimination.

BODY MASS INDEX (BMI) CHART

HEIGHT WEIGHT LB	4'10"	4'11"	5'	5'1"	5'2"	5'3"	5'4"	5'5"	5'6"	5'7"	5'8"
100	20.9	20.2	19.6	18.9	18.3	17.8	17.2	16.7	16.2	15.7	15.2
110	23.0	22.3	21.5	20.8	20.2	19.5	18.9	18.3	17.8	17.3	16.8
120	25.1	24.3	23.5	22.7	22.0	21.3	20.6	20.0	19.4	18.8	18.3
130	27.2	26.3	25.4	24.6	23.8	23.1	22.4	21.7	21.0	20.4	19.8
140	29.3	28.3	27.4	26.5	25.7	24.9	24.1	23.3	22.6	22.0	21.3
150	31.4	30.4	29.4	28.4	27.5	26.6	25.8	25.0	24.3	23.5	22.9
160	33.5	32.4	31.3	30.3	29.3	28.4	27.5	26.7	25.9	25.1	24.4
170	35.6	34.4	33.3	32.2	31.2	30.2	29.2	28.3	27.5	26.7	25.9
180	37.7	36.4	35.2	34.1	33.0	32.0	31.0	30.0	29.1	28.3	27.4
190	39.8	38.5	37.2	36.0	34.8	33.7	32.7	31.7	30.7	29.8	28.9
200	41.9	40.5	39.1	37.9	36.7	35.5	34.4	33.4	32.3	31.4	30.5
205	42.9	41.5	40.1	38.8	37.6	36.4	35.3	34.2	33.2	32.2	31.2
210	44.0	42.5	41.1	39.8	38.5	37.3	36.1	35.0	34.0	33.0	32.0
215	45.0	43.5	42.1	40.7	39.4	38.2	37.0	35.9	34.8	33.7	32.8
220	46.1	44.5	43.1	41.7	40.3	39.1	37.8	36.7	35.6	34.5	33.5
225	47.1	45.5	44.0	42.6	41.2	39.9	38.7	37.5	36.4	35.3	34.3
230	48.2	46.6	45.0	43.5	42.2	40.8	39.6	38.4	37.2	36.1	35.0
235	49.2	47.6	46.0	44.5	43.1	41.7	40.4	39.2	38.0	36.9	35.8
240	50.3	48.6	47.0	45.4	44.0	42.6	41.3	40.0	38.8	37.7	36.6
245	51.3	49.6	47.9	46.4	44.9	43.5	42.1	40.9	39.6	38.5	37.3
250	52.4	50.6	48.9	47.3	45.8	44.4	43.0	41.7	40.4	39.2	38.1
255	53.4	51.6	49.9	48.3	46.7	45.3	43.9	42.5	41.2	40.0	38.9
260	54.5	52.6	50.9	49.2	47.7	46.2	44.7	43.4	42.1	40.8	38.6
265	55.5	53.6	51.9	50.2	48.6	47.0	45.6	44.2	42.9	41.6	40.4
270	56.5	54.6	52.8	51.1	49.5	47.9	46.4	45.0	43.7	42.4	41.1
275	57.6	55.7	53.8	52.1	50.4	48.8	47.3	45.9	44.5	43.2	41.9
280	58.6	56.7	54.8	53.0	51.3	49.7	48.2	46.7	45.3	43.9	42.7
285	59.7	57.7	55.8	54.0	52.2	50.6	49.0	47.5	46.1	44.7	43.4
290	60.7	58.7	56.8	54.9	53.2	51.5	49.9	48.4	46.9	45.5	44.2
295	61.8	59.7	57.7	55.9	54.1	52.4	50.7	49.2	47.7	46.3	44.9
300	62.8	60.7	58.7	56.8	55.0	53.3	51.6	50.0	48.5	47.1	45.7

BODY MASS INDEX (BMI) CHART

5'9"	5'10"	5'11"	6'	6'1"	6'2"	6'3"	6'4"	6'5"	6'6"	6'7"	6'8"
14.8	14.4	14.0	13.6	13.2	12.9	12.5	12.2	11.9	11.6	11.3	11.0
16.3	15.8	15.4	14.9	14.5	14.2	13.8	13.4	13.1	12.7	12.4	12.1
17.8	17.3	16.8	16.3	15.9	15.4	15.0	14.6	14.3	13.9	13.5	13.2
19.2	18.7	18.2	17.7	17.2	16.7	16.3	15.9	15.4	15.1	14.7	14.3
20.7	20.1	19.6	19.0	18.5	18.0	17.5	17.1	16.6	16.2	15.8	15.4
22.2	21.6	21.0	20.4	19.8	19.3	18.8	18.3	17.8	17.4	16.9	16.5
23.7	23.0	22.4	21.7	21.2	20.6	20.0	19.5	19.0	18.5	18.1	17.6
25.2	24.4	23.8	23.1	22.5	21.9	21.3	20.7	20.2	19.7	19.2	18.7
26.6	25.9	25.2	24.5	23.8	23.2	22.5	22.0	21.4	20.8	20.3	19.8
28.1	27.3	26.6	25.8	25.1	24.4	23.8	23.2	22.6	22.0	21.4	20.9
29.6	28.8	28.0	27.2	26.4	25.7	25.1	24.4	23.8	23.2	22.6	22.0
30.3	29.5	28.7	27.9	27.1	26.4	25.7	25.0	24.4	23.7	23.1	22.6
31.1	30.2	29.4	28.5	27.8	27.0	26.3	25.6	25.0	24.3	23.7	23.1
31.8	30.9	30.0	29.2	28.4	27.7	26.9	26.2	25.5	24.9	24.3	23.7
32.6	31.6	30.7	29.9	29.1	28.3	27.6	26.8	26.1	25.5	24.8	24.2
33.3	32.4	31.4	30.6	29.7	28.9	28.2	27.4	26.7	26.1	25.4	24.8
34.0	33.1	32.1	31.3	30.4	29.6	28.8	28.1	27.3	26.6	26.0	25.3
34.8	33.8	32.8	31.9	31.1	30.2	29.4	28.7	27.9	27.2	26.5	25.9
35.5	34.5	33.5	32.6	31.7	30.9	30.1	29.3	28.5	27.8	27.1	26.4
36.3	35.2	34.2	33.3	32.4	31.5	30.7	29.9	29.1	28.4	27.7	27.0
37.0	35.9	34.9	34.0	33.1	32.2	31.3	30.5	29.7	29.0	28.2	27.5
37.7	36.7	35.6	34.7	33.7	32.8	31.9	31.1	30.3	29.5	28.8	28.1
38.5	37.4	36.3	35.3	34.4	33.5	32.6	31.7	30.9	30.1	29.4	28.6
39.2	38.1	37.0	36.0	35.0	34.1	33.2	32.3	31.5	30.7	29.9	29.2
40.0	38.8	37.7	36.7	35.7	34.7	33.8	32.9	32.1	31.3	30.5	29.7
40.7	39.5	38.4	37.4	36.4	35.4	34.4	33.5	32.7	31.8	31.0	30.3
41.4	40.3	39.1	38.1	37.0	36.0	35.0	34.3	33.3	32.4	31.6	30.8
42.2	41.0	39.8	38.7	37.7	36.7	35.7	34.8	33.9	33.0	32.2	31.4
42.9	41.7	40.5	39.4	38.3	37.3	36.3	35.4	34.5	33.6	32.7	31.9
43.7	42.4	41.2	40.1	39.0	38.0	36.9	36.0	35.1	34.2	33.3	32.5
44.4	43.1	41.9	40.8	39.7	38.6	37.6	36.6	35.6	34.7	33.9	33.0

There are so many benefits to losing pounds and to achieving and maintaining a healthy weight, but the majority of people find it very difficult to do so. One reason is that they want an easy solution: a quick fix or magic pill that will make their weight melt away. Another is that often they do not understand all the factors that may be contributing to their weight problem.

WHY PEOPLE ARE OVERWEIGHT OR OBESE

"You're fat because you eat too much." Oh, if it were only that simple. At the most basic level, the reason the majority of people are overweight is that they consume more calories than they burn. However, there are many factors that can cause the imbalance between the number of calories people consume and the amount they use. Those factors include, among others:

- Metabolic rate—the rate at which the body burns calories
- Age
- Heredity/genetics
- Lack of adequate exercise
- Medication—some drugs promote weight gain by slowing metabolism or stimulating appetite
- Nutritional deficiencies—low levels of some nutrients (i.e., vitamins B_6 and B_{12}) hinder fat metabolism or cause depression, which can lead to weight gain
- Psychological factors, such as low self-esteem, use of food as security, and other emotional influences

Except for age, you can influence or change each of the other factors. You can remedy nutritional deficiencies, for example, by changing your eating habits and taking supplements. You can identify which medications may be contributing to weight gain and find alternatives, and if you have a poor self-image, you can seek help from therapists or other emotional support sources.

Another factor that draws a lot of debate is set point. According to Xavier Pi-Sunyer, M.D., director of the Obesity

Research Center at St. Luke's Roosevelt Hospital in New York, when people gain weight and remain at that weight for a length of time, the body sets up a defense system to maintain that weight at all costs. That weight becomes the set point.

The body's defense mechanism has several components. First, in response to a reduction in calories, the metabolic rate declines. Second, as fat cells shrink, they hold onto their contents more readily. Both of these reactions to dieting are survival strategies for the body, but they are frustrating for people who want to lose weight. "The body is very good at defending itself from the danger of being underweight," says Dr. Pi-Sunyer, "but is not really equipped to handle being overweight." That's because over the millennia, people generally have not had a problem with having too much food to eat. "That's a modern problem," says Pi-Sunyer.

And yes, you can even have an impact on your heredity. Researchers believe genes are about one-third responsible for determining a person's weight. One of the ways scientists explored this idea was to study identical twins. They found that even when twins were raised apart in entirely different environments, they tended to have very similar weights.

Yet the remaining two-thirds can be attributed to other factors, including choice of diet, exercise, and the items in the preceding list, which means you *can* influence your weight, even if you are biologically predisposed to being overweight. This is dramatically demonstrated by the Pima Indians of the Southwestern United States and northern Mexico. The Pima are unfortunate enough to be genetically prone to obesity and its complications: about half of adult Pima in Arizona suffer from diabetes caused by obesity. However, their genetically similar cousins in Mexico are thin and diabetes is not a problem among them. So genes may predispose to obesity, but sedentary living and cheap, plentiful, rich food are still necessary to bring it on. Genes are not destiny!

Within the area of heredity and weight, scientists have looked at the genes that control metabolism and appetite. One of these genes determines how much of a certain enzyme called LPL, or lipoprotein lipase, is produced. This enzyme is important because it helps to store calories as fat. If levels of LPL are high, the body is especially efficient at storing excess calories as fat. Researchers at Cedars Sinai Medical Center in Los Angeles found an interesting way in which LPL acts in obese people. In a study of nine obese individuals who lost an average of 90 pounds, LPL levels increased after weight loss, and the more overweight the people were at the beginning of the study, the higher the LPL levels were after they lost the weight. The researchers believe that the body "fights" to regain the weight, and that the gene that controls LPL is activated by weight loss. Ways to control or reduce LPL levels are under study.

HOW TO LOSE WEIGHT

Carolyn Costin, director of the Eating Disorder Center of California, in Malibu, and author of *The Dieting Daughter*, offers basic, sound advice to anyone who is about to embark on a weight-loss program. "Don't do anything to lose weight that you're not prepared to do for the rest of your life, because going on a diet certainly implies that you'll ultimately go off it."

Take a moment to consider what these words mean. What comes to mind when you think about losing weight? Hunger? Depriving yourself of favorite foods? Boring exercises? These are negative, self-defeating thoughts that flash a big message: DANGER AHEAD. YOU ARE ABOUT TO SUFFER. It's no wonder that the vast majority of diets fail.

Losing weight involves positively redesigning your lifestyle, which results in behaviors and goals you can live with for the rest of your life. It's not about deprivation; it's about health, energy, self-esteem, and personal growth. To lose weight in a healthy way and keep it off, consider your attitude about yourself, your weight, and your lifestyle. You are not just your body; you are also mind and spirit, and all three entities work together to create who you are. Therefore, remember to nurture each aspect of yourself when you are redesigning your lifestyle.

Before you start any weight-loss diet plan, you should get a complete physical examination, including a general blood biochemistry panel, and an electrocardiogram if you are older than forty-five. A thorough examination will identify factors that may be contributing to being overweight, such as vitamin and mineral deficiencies or low thyroid function. Make sure to tell your health-care professional about any medications, herbs, or nutrients you are taking.

- Eat nutritious, balanced meals.
- Exercise regularly.
- Develop a loving relationship with yourself and your world.
- Be informed about, not fooled by, weight-loss aids.

It is not the role of this book to provide comprehensive information about the first three guidelines, so coverage here will be brief. There are a wealth of books, articles, and Web sites that can help you. See the Suggested Readings (pp. 191–92) for a sample.

CHOOSE NUTRITIOUS, FRIENDLY FOODS

The secret to losing weight is to create an eating plan that includes a wide variety of foods that are nutritious and that you can live with the rest of your life. To accomplish this, you will probably have to make some changes to your current diet—maybe even some drastic changes—but the transitions will be well worth it. Food should be your friend, not your enemy. Choose foods from different cultures or learn to prepare old favorites in healthy ways.

A mistake many people make is, rather than create a reasonable food plan, they latch onto fad diets or gimmicks. If you starve yourself, you'll lose some weight, but you can't continue to live on a starvation diet. Your health will suffer, and chances are you'll regain all the weight you lost . . . and even more . . . once you begin to eat "normally" again.

A grapefruit diet may help you lose a few pounds fast, but can you really live on grapefruit forever? Some people say they have lost weight eating lots of protein, like steaks, milk, and hamburgers, but have they considered the long-term effects of all that protein on their kidneys and bones, not to mention the fat clogging their arteries and the pesticides and hormones in the animal products? Fads can ruin your health; nutritious, friendly foods can save it.

THE "E" WORD

Exercise is a critical part of any weight-loss program, because it not only keeps your metabolic rate up, it also helps keep muscles toned. When you replace fat with lean muscle, it means a higher metabolism rate. You will look better and feel better, both physically and emotionally. Feeling good about yourself, giving yourself positive affirmations, drawing on the support of friends and relatives, reaching out to others and doing volunteer work, communing with nature—all of these things help build and support your emotional and spiritual foundation, which is also important when you are engaged in a weight-loss program.

LIKING YOUR SELVES

Some people believe that if they could just lose 10 or 20 pounds, their lives would be so much better. They would have more friends, a better job, be more successful, and be happier. But happiness and success are not "out there"; they are inside you. How do you cultivate balance, peace, and harmony within yourself? How can you expand your inner horizons and learn to like all your selves?

Examine your reasons for wanting to lose weight. If your weight is negatively affecting your health, then your motivation seems clear. And there certainly is nothing wrong with wanting to lose weight because you want to look better. But if you think looking better is going to miraculously improve all aspects of your life, then you are not being realistic. If you are not basically a secure, happy person now, being 20 pounds lighter won't suddenly make you so. Marilyn Monroe, although gorgeous, was tragically insecure throughout her short life.

Balance all aspects of your life. If you are overweight, you probably think about it often. But do not allow it to consume your thoughts. Develop and cultivate other interests. Many people find that if they reach out to others, by volunteering to help a favorite charity or cause, they feel richer, more fulfilled, and more satisfied with themselves. You may choose to explore various spiritual paths, get in touch with nature, learn to meditate or do yoga, take up a musical instrument, or write in a journal. Life goes on as you pursue your weight-loss program. If you concentrate on losing weight and ignore other parts of your life, you will not be happy, even when you lose those extra pounds.

It can be helpful to uncover your relationship with your food and how it affects your eating habits. Most people who are overweight don't eat out of hunger; they eat because they are unhappy, depressed, bored, or angry. To discover your relationship with food, keep an eating diary for a week. Write down what, when, where, and how much you eat, including how you are feeling at the time you are eating. This information can help you understand why you are overweight and allow you to take steps to correct it. Many books can help you explore your relationship with food; among them are *Fattitudes: Beat Self-Defeat and Win Your War with Weight* (2000) by Jeffrey and Norean Wilbert; *The Five Reasons Why We Overeat: How to Develop a Long-Term Weight-Control Plan That's Right for You* (1998) by Cynthia Last; and *Emotional Eating: What You Need to Know Before Starting Another Diet* (1998) by Edward Aramson.

It also helps to be realistic—but not resigned—to what nature has dealt you. Genetics play a role in body size and weight. If a look at your family tree shows a definite pattern of short, overweight, pear-shaped women (weight that settles in the hips and thighs), you are probably predisposed to be pear-shaped as well. However, that does not mean your "pear" can't be a thinner, healthier version. Remember: genetics' role is about one-third; you can influence the rest.

GETTING HELP: WEIGHT-LOSS PRODUCTS

The real heart of a weight-loss plan is food, exercise, and mental/spiritual balance, and how you bring them together in a "doable" life plan that works for you. If you are like most people, you would like some help. And if you are realistic, you know that there is no magic solution that will do all the work for you. But there are some products that can either get you started with your weight-loss program or help keep you on track.

The array of weight-loss products on the market is dizzying, and the information you hear and read about them often brings up more questions than it answers. Have you ever picked up a weight-loss product and asked yourself:

- How do these ingredients help promote weight loss?
- Are the milligrams listed for each ingredient sufficient to promote weight loss, or are any or all of the ingredients simply "fillers" that contribute little or nothing to the product?
- Are there any reliable studies that support the weight-loss claims?
- *Is the product safe?* Will it interact with anything else I may be taking?
- What are the side effects?

When it comes to spending money on diet pills, dietary products, and weight-reducing programs, people are quick to open their wallets: according to the American Dietetic Association, Americans dish out $33 billion a year on such items. And among the most popular types of dietary items purchased are pills, foods, and supplements.

But buying weight-loss supplements and products can be a gamble. On the one hand, consumers can be glad they have a tremendous number of these dietary aids from which to choose, and the media makes sure they are constantly reminded of those choices. On the other hand, much of the information about these products is misleading, inaccurate, and confusing.

To add to the confusion, consumers often read conflicting reports on the effectiveness and dangers of many of these products. In some cases, such as with Pondimin (fenfluramine) and Redux (dexfenfluramine), once glowing promises of weight loss were replaced with reports of serious health risks and the products being removed from the market by the manufacturers at the request of the Food and Drug Administration (FDA). In November 1999, another diet product was scrutinized, the over-the-counter product Triax Metabolic Accelerator, which the FDA claimed contains a dangerous amount of thyroid hormone. The manufacturer, Pharmatech, has stopped distributing the drug.

Adding to the confusion is the fact that there have been very few long-term studies of the effectiveness or potential dangers of many of the over-the-counter dietary products currently on the market. Advertisements for many of these dietary aids can be found in magazines and newspapers; on billboards, television, radio, and the Internet. Although most of these advertisements are alluring and convincing, drawing in their audience with promises of fast, easy weight loss and implying they will achieve happiness and the bodies of their dreams, many of them are short on mentioning side effects or emphasizing the realistic results people can expect. The result is a large population of people who are anxious, even desperate, for diet products that work, yet they are not provided with the tools to make appropriate, educated decisions about the products available to them. How do you search among all the rhetoric surrounding these products to find the kernels of truth? How can you identify effective, safe weight-loss products?

HOW THIS BOOK CAN HELP YOU

This book can help you answer these and other questions about dietary products. Each entry in this book provides information under the following headings. Some of the headings and information vary slightly depending on whether the product is an herb, a prescription drug, an over-the-counter combination product, or a dietary food.

- Product
- Brand Name(s)
- Type/Definition
- Ingredients
- How Sold
- Background/Research
- Product Claims
- Dosage Information
- Side Effects
- Precautions
- Further Information

WEIGHT-LOSS RESEARCH

In some cases, there is little or no reliable information about how a substance works and no research to back up any of the claims made by manufacturers. Sometimes the only "research" data available are testimonial accounts from past and current users who have experienced good results with an herb or product. Some of these items are included in the book because they are on the market and being sold and used by millions of people. The lack of information does not mean these products are good or bad; it simply means you should be told what is known or not known about them.

Very often, the "research" claims touted by manufacturers of weight-loss products is highly suspect. Some of the studies have been conducted solely by the manufacturer, who has a vested interest in presenting results that are positive and ignoring those that are not. Often, studies have been done on animals only, and you have no way of knowing whether the results will carry over to humans. Beware of page after page of "testimonials" from those who have reportedly used the product. "T. J. in Oregon" and "Suzy in New York" are likely the creation of the manufacturer's marketing department.

The type of study is important, too. For example, results of a double-blind, placebo-controlled study are much more valid than those in an open-label, uncontrolled study. In a double-blind study, neither the participants nor the people testing them know whether the subjects are taking the active product or a placebo (an inert substance, often a sugar pill). When people know what they are taking, they can greatly influence the results simply by thinking and believing they will respond in a certain way. This is known as the placebo effect. The placebo effect is one of the main problems with open-label studies. If you know you are taking an herb or drug that is supposed to reduce your appetite, you may convince yourself that your appetite is less, and the true effects of the product will not be tested accurately. This is why scientists prefer double-blind, placebo-controlled trials.

If you are interested in specific products, ask the manufacturers if you can see the research that backs up their claims. If they have nothing to hide, they should be happy to oblige. You can also do your own research, beginning with this book. *The Diet Pill Guide* provides references or actual research results for products for which such information is available.

To keep abreast of the latest developments in weight-loss research and products, be alert to announcements about new studies, findings, and products. Look beyond the headlines and advertising hype. When new study results are announced, find out who funded the study and whether the researchers are financially connected in any way to the product or sponsors. See which publication published the results. Is it a journal in which articles are reviewed by a panel of unbiased experts, or is it a publication put out by the company that makes the product being tested? Often you need to be a detective to track down the truth about diet products. But when it comes to your health, isn't a little detective work worth it?

MISCONCEPTIONS ABOUT HERBAL AND NATURAL SUPPLEMENTS

When you shop for weight-loss products, you will probably see the words "herb" and "natural" on many labels and in advertisements. One misconception people have about these words is that they mean a product is safe. Many herbs, vitamins, and other natural supplements are powerful substances. Any substance should be taken according to prescribed or recommended dosing directions. Taking more than the recommended dosage may result in unpleasant or serious side effects. Ephedra is one such example (see the entry in Part II, pp. 67–70). That's why it is important to be informed about the products you wish to take.

Many people also incorrectly believe that manufacturers of herbs, vitamins, and other natural supplements are required to adhere to the same strict guidelines that producers of over-the-counter and prescription pharmaceutical products must follow. This is not true. The lack of regulation of natural products can make it difficult to identify quality herbal and natural remedies.

To help ease the uncertainty, the federal government passed the Dietary Supplement Health and Education Act in 1994. This act offers some consumer protection by requiring that manufacturers label their supplements with specific information about the ingredients (see Reading Herbal Product Labels, p. 18). However, this does not mean you as a consumer are guaranteed to get what you pay for. Elizabeth Yetley, Ph.D., director of the Food and Drug Administration Office of Special Nutritionals, says that although most supplement manufacturers are "responsible and careful," "consumers need to be discriminating. The FDA and industry have important roles to play, but consumers must take responsibility too." This book helps you take that responsibility into your own hands.

WHAT YOU CAN EXPECT FROM WEIGHT-LOSS PRODUCTS

In the majority of cases, the best you can expect from prescription, OTC, or herbal weight-loss products is a *slight increase in the amount of overall weight you lose* when you use them along with the three basics of weight loss: a sensible, nutritious eating plan, regular exercise, and emotional/spiritual support.

For example, if you and a friend made a pact to eat a healthy, low-calorie diet and to exercise together and you lose 20 pounds, the best you could possibly expect from including a diet product to your plan would be a loss of an additional 2 pounds, or 10 percent of total weight lost. Why? Because weight-loss pills cannot take the place of the three basic essentials for weight loss. There are no miracles in a pill. The miracle must come from within you.

Many remedies do little more than make your wallet lighter. Many weight-loss products are pricey, especially those marketed as "package deals," requiring that you buy the shakes, nutrition bars, special meals, and additional supplements if you want to get results. If you want to consider such plans, it is best to review all the literature about them alone, away from the distributor or salesperson, so you can take the time to honestly ask yourself whether you will follow the plan, whether the cost is reasonable and justifiable, and whether other options would make more sense.

Worse, however, is that weight-loss products can be dangerous. The Food and Drug Administration periodically receives reports of adverse effects, *even deaths*, associated with the use of various weight-loss products. Two of the most notorious products were Pondimin (fenfluramine) and Redux (dexfenfluramine). Fenfluramine was combined by some doctors with phentermine in the popular diet drug combo known as fen-phen. Fenfluramine and dexfenfluramine were withdrawn from the marketplace by the manufacturer in 1997. The other half of the fen-phen combination drug—phentermine—was determined to be safe and is still available as a prescription weight-loss product. Redux and Pondimin use was associated with several problems, the most serious of which was a greater chance of getting pulmonary hypertension when taking the drug. This is a rare and potentially fatal disease that usually affects women aged thirty to fifty years, perhaps the biggest market for diet products. Around the same time, researchers found that some people who were taking fen-phen or Redux were developing heart abnormalities. After more than 100 cases of heart-valve problems were detected, both Redux and Pondimin were pulled from the market.

Another weight-loss product that is still controversial is ephedra, also known as ma huang. This herbal product has been linked with more than 60 deaths and over 800 medical complaints. In a recent case (May 2000), for example, a thirty-four-year-old man suffered a stroke after taking a product containing ephedra. Many states now ban or restrict the sale of ephedra or products containing it. You can read more about the dangers of ephedra in Part II of this book.

The take-home message is be informed. Weight-loss products are a multibillion-dollar business. They also are products that command much emotion from those who buy them, and they have the potential to harm people's health. Thus the use of weight-loss products is not something you should enter into lightly, for several reasons: both individual substances and combination products can be unsafe, you may not get the desired results, and you can waste time and money. Each of these reasons boils down to one thing: theft of your health, your trust, and your lifestyle. Take control of what you put into your body, and you will be better for it.

READING HERBAL PRODUCT LABELS

Look for the following information when shopping for herbal and nutritional products.

- For herbs: The Latin name, including genus and species, or the common name. Most herbs have more than one species. Make sure you buy the one that has medicinal value. (This means you need to do a little research before going to the store.)
- For herbs: Parts of the plant used. Different plant parts can provide different effects. If you buy fennel, for example, you want the seeds, because they are the part of the plant that may offer the weight-loss benefits.

- Facts about the supplement: This information appears in a box and includes "Serving Size"; "Amount Per Serving" of the herb (usually in milligrams); and "% Daily Value," which will be noted as "Daily Value not Established" in the case of herbs and some nutrients.
- Other ingredients: If possible, buy remedies that are made without fillers, such as talc, cornstarch, wheat, artificial colors, artificial flavors, and artificial preservatives. Capsules can be made of gelatin (an animal by-product) or have a vegetable base. Tablets typically contain ingredients such as magnesium stearate and cellulose, which are used to make the pills and considered to be harmless.
- Expiration date: This date is approximately when the supplement's potency will fall below that stated on the label.
- Recommendations for use: This part of the label explains when and how much of the supplement to take and whether the supplement can be taken by children.
- The amount, form, and potency of the herbal product: For example, a cayenne label may read: "50 capsules, 40,000 HU (heating units), 400 mg each." Buy a product that is convenient to take. If the recommended dose is 400 mg 2 times a day, don't buy 100-mg capsules because you'll need to take 4 capsules for each dose.
- Warning or caution: Limitations of use (for example, do not use if pregnant or breast-feeding) and known side effects. The warning may seem benign, such as "consult your doctor before taking this product" without any specific warnings. However, it is recommended that you do talk with a pharmacist or other health professional before taking weight-loss products, especially if you have any type of medical condition, are taking medication, vitamins, or other supplements, or are elderly.
- A statement about additives: For example—"This product is free of milk, wheat, soy, sugar, salt, and corn." This can be important if you are allergic to these ingredients.

- Storage instructions: Supplements that are stored incorrectly can rapidly lose their potency.
- A statement that tells how the product can maintain healthy or normal structures or functions of the human body: For example—a label for cayenne may say that it is a "blood-red warming herb that has an invigorating effect on several body systems." Such claims *must* be accompanied by the following: "These statements have not been evaluated by the Food and Drug Administration. This product is not intended to diagnose, treat, cure, or prevent any disease."
- Lot number: This often appears on the bottom of the package. This number helps the manufacturer locate the original batch if there is a problem with the product.
- Manufacturer's name and address or toll-free customer service telephone number: Some now supply Web site or E-mail information.
- Organically grown: Because manufacturers cannot always get organically grown herbs, the label may say that organically grown herbs are used "when available."

PART I

Prescription Weight-Loss Drugs

PRESCRIPTION WEIGHT-LOSS drugs can be a blessing and a curse. When they are used by the people for whom they were developed (individuals with medically significant weight problems), along with dietary, behavioral, and exercise programs that are necessary for their success, they can be, literally, a lifesaver. Research shows that even the loss of 5 percent of body weight in obese individuals can make a very significant and positive impact on their health. It greatly reduces the risk of heart disease, diabetes, stroke, and high blood pressure, or at least the symptoms and complications that accompany these conditions. However, many individuals believe diet drugs are magical and will help them lose weight, and keep it off, with little or no effort on their part. Those who accept the responsibility that comes with taking prescription diet medications, which includes eating a reduced-calorie diet, getting regular exercise, and following the manufacturer's recommendations to take the drugs for the *limited prescribed time only*, can expect success. Among those who expect miracles, there can only be disappointment.

WHO IS A CANDIDATE FOR PRESCRIPTION DIET DRUGS?

The manufacturers of prescription diet drugs and the Food and Drug Administration (FDA) are both clear about the medically acceptable use of these medications: they are reserved for individuals who are obese—individuals with a BMI greater than 30, or those with a BMI greater than 27 and associated weight-related problems such as high blood pressure, diabetes, arthritis, and so on. Prescription diet drugs are not recommended for anyone who is mildly overweight. Thus these drugs are not for people who want to lose weight for cosmetic reasons.

WHO IS REALLY TAKING THESE DRUGS?

Unfortunately, many people who do not fit these foregoing criteria are taking prescription diet pills. They are getting them from their doctors, who are succumbing to the demands of their patients; they get them from friends and family members; and they get them illegally.

RISKS ASSOCIATED WITH PRESCRIPTION DIET DRUGS

Prescription weight-loss drugs are powerful, and with power comes risk. Here are some concerns you and your doctor should discuss:

- **Potential for dependence or abuse.** Most prescription diet pills are controlled substances, which means they have the potential for abuse and dependence. (See the box for a definition of controlled substances, p. 24.) Not all of the drugs are in the same classification, and your doctor should discuss any risks that are especially relevant for you.
- **Tolerance.** Most prescription diet drugs suppress the appetite. After taking appetite-suppressant drugs for several months, weight loss tends to stop, even if patients continue to take the drug, and in many cases patients begin to gain back weight. It is not yet clear whether this means patients have developed a tolerance to the medication or whether the drug has reached the

limit of its effectiveness. In either case, the result is the same: the vast majority of people begin to gain back the weight they lost during the first few months on the prescription medication.

- **Side effects.** Any substance people ingest can cause side effects: even something as benign as water, if you drink it to excess, can cause bloating and stomach pain or even abnormalities of blood chemistry. But prescription diet pills are associated with a wide range of adverse reactions, some of which can be severe and life-threatening. You will find a list of side effects with each entry. You should discuss these with your physician before you decide to take diet drugs. If you have friends or relatives who have taken the drug you are considering, talk to them as well. It is helpful to know the types of experiences you may expect.

Your doctor should conduct a thorough medical evaluation before deciding if you are a candidate for prescription diet drugs. The degree of obesity (your body mass index, or BMI; see the Introduction); your personal and family medical history; current health status; use of other medications; past and current use of alcohol; and methods of weight loss you have used in the past should all be considered in the evaluation. Blood pressure and blood tests also should be done. Even if you fit the criterion for obesity, you may not be eligible for prescription medication because of contraindications in any of these areas; for example, if you have a heart condition or a history of substance abuse. Fortunately, there are other dietary aids you can consider; they are discussed in Parts II and III of this book.

Some of the drugs in this section are described as nonamphetamine or related to amphetamine drugs. As a point of reference, amphetamines are potent central nervous system stimulants, which eliminate fatigue, suppress appetite, and give you a sense of well-being and alertness. But they are also habit-forming and associated with a long list of effects, including but not limited to dry mouth; nausea; vomiting; diarrhea; heart palpitations; fever; tremors; restlessness; and anxiety.

As always, regardless of whether you and your doctor decide on a prescription medication or any of the other nonprescription dietary aids, the one "prescription" that applies to everyone who wants to lose weight is a reduced-calorie diet and exercise. And because that is often the hardest pill to swallow, you may get a boost from some of the others.

CONTROLLED SUBSTANCES SCHEDULE

Schedule II: High potential for abuse. Currently accepted medical use in the U.S.; abuse may lead to severe psychological or physical dependence.
Schedule III: Potential for abuse less than II; well-documented and accepted medical use in the U.S.; abuse may lead to moderate or low physical dependence or high psychological dependence.
Schedule IV: Low potential for abuse; limited physical and/or psychological dependence.

Benzphetamine

BRAND NAME(S): Didrex.
TYPE/DEFINITION: An appetite suppressant that is chemically related to amphetamines. It is a schedule III controlled substance, with moderate potential for abuse.
HOW SOLD: Benzphetamine is available in 25-mg and 50-mg immediate-release tablets and 75-mg controlled-release tablets. The tablets also contain inactive ingredients: calcium stearate, cornstarch; ervthrosine sodium; FD 8 C yellow No. 61; lactose; providone; sorbitol.
RESEARCH: Benzphetamine was approved for weight management by the Food and Drug Administration in 1960; therefore most of the research studies are quite dated. One of the early

studies was published in *Drugs*, in which benzphetamine was identified as an addictive substance. Other studies, many of which were conducted in Europe, substantiated its usefulness as a weight-loss aid when combined with a low-calorie diet and exercise. These and others studies are listed in Further Information.

PRODUCT CLAIMS: Benzphetamine stimulates the satiety (feeling of fullness) center in the hypothalamus and limbic regions of the brain, where appetite and hunger are controlled. When benzphetamine is used along with a low-calorie diet, behavior modification, and a regular exercise program, it can increase the amount of weight lost by about 10 percent. However, weight loss may be temporary only, especially after the drug is discontinued. To maintain weight loss or to continue to lose additional weight after stopping benzphetamine, it is necessary to follow a sensible eating plan and an exercise program.

DOSAGE INFORMATION: Treatment should be individualized and determined by your physician, based on your needs. Benzphetamine can be taken as a single 75-mg (sustained release) dose in midmorning or midafternoon, or the regular tablets (25- or 50-mg) can be taken on an empty stomach 1 hour before meals. Maximum dosage is 150 mg per day.

Do not take a double dose. If you miss a dose and it is almost time for your next one or it is late afternoon or later, skip the missed dose and wait until your next scheduled dose.

SIDE EFFECTS: The most common side effects include nervousness; irritability; headache; sweating; dry mouth; nausea; insomnia; and constipation. Some individuals experience palpitations and an increase in blood pressure.

PRECAUTIONS: Do not take benzphetamine if you are also taking an MAO inhibitor or any central nervous system stimulants; or if you have any of the following conditions: arteriosclerosis, or hardening of the arteries; cardiovascular disease; hypertension; glaucoma; or hyperthyroidism. Do not use this drug if you are or may become pregnant, as it can harm the fetus. Abuse of benzphetamine can cause psychological dependence and severe social dysfunction.

Benzphetamine, like other appetite suppressants, often causes dry mouth, which can increase the chance of developing gum disease and dental cavities. Special attention to oral hygiene, including use of sugarless gum and sugarless hard candies, or sucking on ice chips, is recommended while taking this drug.

FURTHER INFORMATION: **Print:** Craddock, D., Anorectic drugs: Use in general practice. *Drugs*, 1976, 11(5): 378–93; Linquette, A., and Fossati, P., Hunger control with benzphetamine hydrochloride in the treatment of obesity. *Lille Med*, Apr. 1971, 16(Suppl 2): 620–24; Plauchu, M. et al., Trial of benzphetamine in treatment of obesity. *Lyon Med*, Sept. 14, 1969, 222(32): 317–21; Wynn, R. L., Dental considerations of patients taking appetite suppressants. *Gen Den*, Jul.–Aug. 1997, 45 (4): 324–28. **Web site:** www.weightloss2000.com.

Diethylpropion hydrochloride

BRAND NAME(S): Depletite, Depletite LA, Tenuate Dospan, Tepanil; generic available.

TYPE/DEFINITION: Diethylpropion is an appetite suppressant, sympathomimetic (causes a rise in blood pressure and a slowing of the heart rate), and central nervous system stimulant. It was approved for weight management by the Food and Drug Administration in 1959 and is a schedule IV controlled substance, with low potential for abuse.

HOW SOLD: Diethylpropion is available as 25-mg tablets (immediate release) and 75-mg tablets (sustained release).

RESEARCH: In a double-blind, placebo-controlled study, patients taking diethylpropion hydrochloride lost an average of 1.32 pounds per week compared with patients on placebo, who lost 0.84 pounds per week. At the end of the 12-week study, those who had taken diethylpropion lost an average of 15.9 pounds compared with 10.0 pounds for those taking placebo. The researcher noted that "amphetamine-like side effects were virtually absent." However, amphetamine-like side effects, including those listed below ("Side Effects"), are commonly associated with this drug.

The findings were similar in another double-blind, placebo-controlled study. Researchers in New Zealand found that patients who took diethylpropion had significantly more weight loss than those who took placebo and that the side effects experienced by the drug-treated group were not significantly greater than those suffered by participants in the placebo group.

PRODUCT CLAIMS: Diethylpropion stimulates the satiety (feeling of fullness) center in the hypothalamus and limbic regions of the brain, where appetite and hunger are controlled. Because diethylpropion has amphetamine-like qualities, it has the potential to cause psychological dependency. This product can be effective as a weight-loss agent if it is used along with a low-calorie diet, behavior modification, and a regular exercise program. However, weight loss may be only temporary, especially after the drug is discontinued. To maintain weight loss or to continue to lose additional weight after stopping diethylpropion, it is necessary to follow a sensible eating plan and an exercise program.

DOSAGE INFORMATION: Diethylpropion is indicated for short-term use (no longer than 12 weeks) for treatment of exogenous obesity (obesity caused by excess intake of calories). It is not indicated for cosmetic weight loss. If you are younger than sixty years, take a 25-mg immediate release tablet 3 times daily 1 hour before meals. For the sustained release, take a 75-mg tablet 10 to 14 hours before bedtime. If you are sixty years or older, you may need to reduce the dosage. Consult with your physician before you start taking this drug. Do not give to children younger than 12 years.

If you miss a dose, take the missed dose as soon as possible unless it is nearly time for your next one. In that case, skip the missed dose and continue with your regular schedule.

SIDE EFFECTS: Common side effects include irritability and insomnia. Less common ones include anxiety; blurred vision; changes in libido; dry mouth; dysphoria (mood of restlessness, dissatisfaction, unhappiness); dizziness; euphoria; headache; hypertension; irregular or pounding heartbeat; nausea or vomiting; rash; sweating; and tremor.

PRECAUTIONS: Diethylpropion should not be used by individuals who are allergic to the drug or by those who have a history of arteriosclerosis or hardening of the arteries; glaucoma; high blood pressure; cardiovascular disease; pulmonary hypertension; hyperthyroidism; alcohol or drug abuse; arrhythmias; kidney or thyroid disease; mental illness; or epilepsy. In particular, diethylpropion can dramatically increase blood pressure and the risk of stroke when combined with phenelazine (Nardil), tranylcypromine (Parnate), or furazolidone (Furazolidone).

Diethylpropion also should not be taken by anyone who has taken drugs of the MAO inhibitor class within the last 2 weeks or an anorectic substance within the last year. If you are taking any of the following substances, consult your doctor before starting diethylpropion: amantadine; amphetamines; any medications for hyperactivity; any appetite-control drugs; chlophedianol; asthma medications, prescription or OTC decongestants or antihistamines; methylphenidate; nabilone; and pemoline. Do not take any other type of anorectic substance, including prescription, over-the-counter, or herbal product while taking diethylpropion. Avoid all foods, beverages, and medications that contain caffeine while taking diethylpropion. Inform your physician and dentist that you are taking diethylpropion before you undergo any type of treatment.

Diethylpropion has the potential to be addictive. If tolerance develops, gradually discontinue use while under the supervision of your doctor. Do not operate a motor vehicle or heavy machinery when taking this drug if you feel drowsy.

This drug should not be taken for longer than 3 months. Longer use has been associated with an increase in the risk of developing pulmonary hypertension, a rare but fatal illness.

No adequate studies have been done in pregnancy, therefore do not use diethylpropion if you are pregnant or think you might be. Weight loss during pregnancy, even for obese persons, is not appropriate as it can harm the fetus. It is not known whether diethylpropion is secreted in breast milk, thus it is best not to use this drug while breast-feeding.

Diethylpropion, like other appetite suppressants, often causes dry mouth, which can increase the chance of developing gum disease and dental cavities. Special attention to oral hygiene, including use of sugarless gum and sugarless hard candies, or sucking on ice chips, is recommended while taking these drugs.

FURTHER INFORMATION: **Print:** Elliott, B. J., A double-blind controlled study of the use of diethylpropion hydrochloride (Tenuate) in obese patients in a rural practice. *New Zealand Med J*, Oct. 25, 1978, 88 (622): 321–322; Parsons, W. B., Jr., Controlled-release diethylpropion hydrochloride used in a program for weight reduction. *Clinical Therapeutics*, 1981; 3 (5): 329–35.

Fluoxetine

BRAND NAME(S): Prozac.
TYPE/DEFINITION: Fluoxetine is an antidepressant, specifically a selective serotonin reuptake inhibitor (SSRI), which has FDA approval for treatment of depression, bulimia, and obsessive-compulsive disorder. Many physicians, however, prescribe it for weight loss, which is considered to be an off-label use. Off-label use refers to use that is not approved by the FDA or included or disclaimed on the approved labeling, but it does not imply improper or illegal use.
HOW SOLD: Available in capsules, 10 mg and 20 mg; preparation also available as a liquid.
RESEARCH: In 1999, a study by researchers at Columbia University in New York City found that fluoxetine reduced food intake for about 4 months in nondepressed obese individuals. Unfortunately, the participants regained the weight they lost during the first few weeks of the study, even when their calorie intake remained low. These results seemed to confirm the earlier findings by Lilly. However, Lilly is now developing a related compound, R-fluoxetine, for additional uses, including

obesity. This fluoxetine product may be classified as an obesity medication by the year 2003 or sooner.

PRODUCT CLAIMS: Researchers are not certain exactly why fluoxetine may help people lose weight. Some experts believe its antidepressant action helps people who tend to overeat when they are depressed. Others say it reduces appetite or raises the metabolic rate. Further studies are needed to make this determination.

DOSAGE INFORMATION: Fluoxetine should only be taken while you are under the medical supervision of your physician. The typical dosage for obesity is 20 mg taken 3 times daily. Initial doses may be less, with a gradual buildup to 20 mg per dose. Older individuals should start with lower doses of 5 mg per day. Total daily intake for all individuals should not exceed 80 mg.

SIDE EFFECTS: The most common side effects are fatigue; diarrhea; sweating; headache; insomnia; vomiting; nausea; thirst; and impaired sexual function.

PRECAUTIONS: People who have diabetes, seizure disorders, renal or liver problems, or who are at risk for suicide should not take fluoxetine. Fluoxetine reacts with other medications by either increasing or decreasing the effects of those drugs, including but not limited to: lithium; diazepam; trazodone; carbamazepine; hydantoin; and tricyclics. Alcohol should be avoided while taking fluoxetine.

FURTHER INFORMATION: There is little information about the use of fluoxetine solely as a weight-loss product. **Print:** Ward, A. S. et al., Fluoxetine-maintained obese humans: effect on food intake and body weight. *Physiol Behav*, July 1999, 66(5): 815–21.

Mazindol

BRAND NAME(S): Mazanor, Sanorex.

TYPE/DEFINITION: A nonamphetamine appetite suppressant, schedule IV controlled substance with low potential for abuse. Mazindol was approved for weight management by the Food and Drug Administration in 1973.

HOW SOLD: Mazindol is available in 1- and 2-mg tablets.

RESEARCH: Many studies have looked at the effectiveness and safety of mazindol. Several of those studies are listed under Further Information. In a Japanese study published in 1995, the average amount of weight lost was about 15 pounds when mazindol was used along with a very-low-calorie diet. About 53 percent of the patients kept the weight off after stopping the very-low-calorie diet, at least for a short time. The patients also had improved cholesterol, triglyceride, and blood pressure levels. These additional benefits have been seen in other studies as well.

Because it is difficult for people to continue to lose weight after being on a very-low-calorie diet and then going off of it, researchers looked at whether mazindol could help in these situations. In 1996, Japanese researchers tested their theory in thirteen severely obese women. They found that mazindol resulted in additional weight loss averaging 15 pounds after 3 months of treatment. The women also had improved insulin sensitivity associated with mazindol use, which resulted in relatively stable blood sugar and energy levels.

One recent study (1997) noted that two men experienced a semenlike discharge while taking mazindol. This adverse reaction was not listed with the expected side effects, and the researchers suggested that it be added to the list of adverse effect possibilities.

PRODUCT CLAIMS: Mazindol stimulates the satiety (feeling of fullness) center in the hypothalamus and limbic regions of the brain, where appetite and hunger are controlled. To be effective, mazindol must be used along with a low-calorie eating plan, behavior modification, and a regular exercise program. However, weight loss may be only temporary, especially after the drug is discontinued. To maintain weight loss or to continue to lose additional weight after stopping mazindol, it is necessary to follow a sensible eating plan and an exercise program.

DOSAGE INFORMATION: Mazindol should be used only under a doctor's supervision and for no longer than 2 to 3 months. The typical dose is 1 mg 3 times per day, 1 hour before meals; or 2 mg 1 time per day, before lunch. If stomach upset occurs, you can take it after meals.

SIDE EFFECTS: Although mazindol is not an amphetamine, it causes many of the same side effects, including nervousness; restlessness; insomnia; euphoria; and overstimulation. Less common side effects include high blood pressure; heart palpitations; drowsiness or sedation; dizziness; tremors; headache; dry mouth; nausea; vomiting; diarrhea; rash; itching; hair loss; muscle pain; sweating; chills; blurred vision; fever; changes in sex drive; urinary retention; testicular pain; and weakness.

PRECAUTIONS: Do not take mazindol if you have high blood pressure, thyroid disease, glaucoma, or heart disease, or if you are sensitive or allergic to any type of appetite suppressant—prescription or nonprescription. Avoid mazindol if you are prone to substance abuse, emotional agitation, or have suicidal thoughts. Older individuals should not take mazindol unless under a doctor's strict supervision.

Mazindol can interact with other medications. Because mazindol stimulates the brain and nerves, if it is taken along with other stimulants such as cold remedies, decongestants, and some asthma medicines, it can raise blood pressure and heart rate. Mazindol should not be taken within 14 days of any MAO inhibitor, as it may result in extremely high blood pressure. If you are taking high blood pressure medication, mazindol may reduce the effects of the medication.

Mazindol, like other appetite suppressants, often causes dry mouth, which can increase the chance of developing gum disease and dental cavities. Special attention to oral hygiene, including use of sugarless gum and sugarless hard candies, drinking lots of water, or sucking on ice chips, is recommended while taking these drugs.

Research shows that large doses of mazindol can harm the fetus. Do not use mazindol if you are pregnant or could be pregnant. Because it is not known whether mazindol passes into breast milk, women who are breast-feeding should not take mazindol.

FURTHER INFORMATION: **Print:** Dolecek, R., Endocrine studies with mazindol in obese patients. *Pharmatherapeutica*, 1980, 2(5): 309–16; Inoue, S., Clinical studies with mazindol. *Obes Res*, Nov. 1995, 3(Suppl 4): 549S–552S; Nishikawa, T. et al., Effect of mazindol on body weight and insulin sensitivity in severely obese patients after a very-low-calorie diet therapy. *Endocr J*, Dec. 1996, 43(6): 671–77; Stall, K. A. and Imperiale, T. F., An overview of the efficacy and safety of fenfluramine and mazindol in the treatment of obesity. *Arch Fam Med*, Oct. 1993, 2(10) 1033–38; van Purjenbroek, E. P., and Meyboom, R. H. Semen-like urethral discharge during the use of mazindol. *Int J Eat Disord*, Jul. 1998, 24(1): 111–13; Yoshida, T. et al. Usefulness of mazindol in combined diet therapy consisting of a low-calorie diet and Optifast in severely obese women. *Int J Clin Pharmacol Res*, 1994, 14(4): 125–32.

Orlistat

BRAND NAME(S): Xenical.
TYPE/DEFINITION: Orlistat works on the digestive system, where it blocks absorption of about one-third of the fat in the food you eat. Orlistat was approved by the Food and Drug Administration on April 26, 1999.
HOW SOLD: Orlistat is available in 120-mg capsules.
RESEARCH: According to the FDA, before orlistat hit the market, it was tested in seven clinical trials (the European Multicentre Orlistat Study) in which more than 4,000 obese people participated. In each case, orlistat was used along with a low-calorie, low-fat diet and regular exercise. Overall, 57 percent of people taking orlistat lost at least 5 percent of their original body weight, compared to 31 percent of participants who took placebos. In one study, people who took orlistat lost an average of 22.7 pounds compared with 13.4 pounds among people who took placebos. Results of a two-year study show that participants who followed a weight-loss plan for 1 year and then switched to a weight-maintenance plan for another year regained some of the weight they lost, even though they contin-

ued to take orlistat. Those who continued to take the drug, however, regained less weight than people who did not take orlistat.

The investigators with the European Multicentre Orlistat Study Group concluded that orlistat is effective for weight control when used along with a calorie-controlled diet in people who are at high risk for hypertension, type II diabetes, or heart disease. Unlike most weight-loss products, orlistat appears to be effective for long-term use when used in conjunction with a low-calorie diet. However, they emphasize that the use of the drug beyond a 2-year period needs to be carefully monitored.

In May 2000, researchers at St. Luke's–Roosevelt Hospital in New York City reported that orlistat may be useful in the treatment of diabetes. The investigators found that orlistat can reverse high blood-sugar levels and perhaps even prevent type II diabetes in obese individuals when it is taken along with a conventional weight-loss program. (This study was supported by the manufacturer of orlistat, Hoffman–La Roche.)

Several trials showed an increased frequency of breast cancer among female users. However, after reevaluating the data, researchers decided that given that breast cancer typically takes years to develop, and based on the size of the tumors and the length of time the patients had been taking the medication, the tumors had been present before the study had started. Therefore, use of orlistat does not appear to induce tumors.

PRODUCT CLAIMS: Unlike other anti-obesity products, which work in the brain, orlistat works on the gastrointestinal tract. It inhibits the action of an enzyme called lipase, which is found in the intestinal tract. Lipase breaks down dietary fat so the body can absorb it. Orlistat blocks absorption of up to 30 percent of dietary fat, allowing the unabsorbed fat to be eliminated in the stool. Because only about 1 percent of orlistat enters the bloodstream, it does not affect the rest of the body and should be safe.

DOSAGE INFORMATION: The FDA recommends that orlistat be taken only by people with a BMI of 30 or greater, or by those with a BMI of 27 or greater if they also have high blood pressure, diabetes, or high cholesterol. The typical dose is 120 mg 3 times daily with meals or up to 1 hour after eating meals that contain fat. Orlistat should be used along with a reduced-calorie diet that contains no more than 30 percent of calories from fat. *If a meal does not contain fat or you skip a meal, do not take the drug.*

SIDE EFFECTS: Users may experience oily rectal seepage, fecal urgency, gas with discharge, and frequent, oily bowel movements. These side effects worsen as dietary fat intake increases, but decrease as dietary fat intake decreases. Orlistat also interferes with the absorption of fat-soluble vitamins, which include vitamins A, D, E, and K, as well as beta-carotene.

PRECAUTIONS: The FDA recommends taking a vitamin supplement that contains the fat-soluble vitamins and beta-carotene 2 hours before or after taking orlistat. Individuals with bulimia nervosa or binge-eating disorders should not take orlistat. Because there are no well-controlled studies of orlistat in pregnancy or breast-feeding, women in these situations should not take the drug.

FURTHER INFORMATION: **Print:** Hollander, P. A., Role of orlistat in the treatment of patients with Type-2 diabetes: A one-year randomized double-blind study. *Diabetes Care*, 1998, 21:1288–1294; Sheen, A. J., Study of the month: Long-term (1–2) years clinical trials with orlistat: a new drug for the treatment of obesity. *Rev Med Liege*, Aug. 1999, 54(8): 707–9; Sheen, A. J., et al., Pharmacy—clinics medication of the month. Orlistat. *Rev Med Liege*, Mar. 1999, 54(3): 192–96; Sjostrom, L. et al., Randomized placebo-controlled trial of orlistat for weight loss and prevention of weight regain in obese patients. *Lancet*, July 18, 1998, 352:167–172. **Web site:** www.xenical.com.

Phentermine (phentermine hydrochloride)

BRAND NAME(S): Adipex-P, Dapex, Fastin, Obe-Nix, Obephen, Obermine, Obestin-30, Ona-Mast, Parmine, Phentrol, T-Diet, Teramin, Unifast Unicelles, Wilpowr.

TYPE/DEFINITION: An appetite suppressant and central nervous system stimulant; formerly part of the combination product fen-phen. Phentermine was approved for weight management by the FDA in 1973. It is a Schedule IV controlled substance, with low potential for abuse.

HOW SOLD: Phentermine is available in 15-mg and 30-mg capsules, and also as phentermine hydrochloride in 37.5-mg. capsules, equivalent to 30 mg of phentermine base.

RESEARCH: Most of the recently published studies of phentermine include its use in combination with fenfluramine. One of the studies in which its effectiveness alone was analyzed found that the drug resulted in an average weight loss of 14 pounds after 20 weeks of treatment.

The biggest concern about use of the combination product fen-phen was the increased risk of heart-valve abnormalities. In the May 2000 issue of *Circulation*, researchers reported on the results of their extensive investigation into this matter, stating that "findings suggest that valvular abnormalities in patients who took fenfluramine-phentermine primarily involve those who had taken these medications for more than 6 months and predominantly results in mild aortic regurgitation." This study did not show the use of phentermine alone to be associated with heart problems. As discussed above, the fen/phen combination was.

PRODUCT CLAIMS: Phentermine stimulates the satiety (feeling of fullness) center in the hypothalamus and limbic regions of the brain, where appetite and hunger are controlled. To be effective, phentermine must be used along with a sensible eating plan, behavior modification, and a regular exercise program. However, weight loss may be temporary only, especially after the drug is discontinued. To maintain weight loss or to continue to lose additional weight after stopping phentermine, it is necessary to follow a sensible eating plan and an exercise program.

DOSAGE INFORMATION: Phentermine can be taken several ways, depending on your lifestyle. One 30-mg capsule decreases appetite for about 12 to 14 hours. (1) Take 1 capsule 30 minutes before breakfast on an empty stomach. Do not take late in the day, as it can make it difficult to fall asleep or stay asleep. (2) Take 1 capsule about 2 hours after breakfast. Phentermine is only approved for use for 12 weeks, after which some users reach drug tolerance and weight loss ceases.

SIDE EFFECTS: The most common side effects include dry mouth; nausea; sleeplessness; headache; stomach upset; constipation; and irritability.

PRECAUTIONS: If you have any of the following medical conditions, tell your doctor before starting phentermine: high blood pressure, overactive thyroid, glaucoma, diabetes, or emotional problems. Limit alcohol use, as it can cause dizziness. Do not take phentermine if you are also taking an MAO inhibitor.

Phentermine, like other appetite suppressants, often causes dry mouth, which can increase the chance of developing gum disease and dental cavities. Special attention to oral hygiene, including use of sugarless gum and sugarless hard candies, drinking lots of water, or sucking on ice chips, is recommended while taking these drugs.

FURTHER INFORMATION: **Print:** Derby, L. E. et al., Use of dexfenfluramine, fenfluramine, and phentermine and the risk of stroke. *Br J Clin Pharmacol*, May 1999, 47(5): 565–69; Douglas, A. et al., Plasma phentermine levels, weight loss and side effects. *Int J Obes*, 1983, 7(6): 591–95; Kokkinos J., and Levine S. R., Possible association of ischemic stroke with phentermine. *Stroke*, Feb. 1993, 24(2): 310–13; Jollis, J. G. et al., Fenfluramine and phentermine and cardiovascular findings: Effect of treatment duration on prevalence of valve abnormalities. *Circulation*, May 2, 2000, 101(17): 2071–77.

Web site: www.rxlist.com/cgi/weight/phenterm/htm.

Phendimetrazine (phendimetrazine tartrate)

BRAND NAME(S): Adipost, Adphen, Anorex, Bacarate, Bontril, Dyrexan-OD, Metra, Obalan, Phenzine, Statobex, Trimstat, Wehhless, and others.

TYPE/DEFINITION: An appetite suppressant and amphetamine-like stimulant. Phendimetrazine was approved for weight management by the Food and Drug Administration in 1961. It is a schedule III controlled substance.

HOW SOLD: Phendimetrazine is available in 35-mg tablets, 35-mg capsules, and 105-mg sustained-release capsules.

RESEARCH/COMMENTS: Phendimetrazine has been in use for about forty years, therefore the majority of the research on this drug is quite dated.

PRODUCT CLAIMS: Phendimetrazine stimulates the satiety (feeling of fullness) center in the hypothalamus and limbic regions of the brain, where appetite and hunger are controlled. There is some evidence that phendimetrazine may temporarily increase the metabolic rate, but this has not been proven. Phendimetrazine can lead to weight loss along with an increase in energy level. However, weight loss may be temporary only, especially after the drug is discontinued. To maintain weight loss or to continue to lose additional weight after stopping phendimetrazine, it is necessary to follow a sensible eating plan and an exercise program.

DOSAGE INFORMATION: The typical dose is a 35-mg tablet or capsule 3 times daily before meals, or a 105-mg sustained-release capsule before lunch. To avoid sleeping problems, take the regular tablets 4 to 6 hours before bedtime or the sustained capsules 10 to 14 hours before you retire. Because drug tolerance develops within 3 to 12 weeks, phendimetrazine should not be taken for longer than 3 months.

If you miss a dose, take the missed dose as soon as possible unless it is nearly time for your next one. In that case, skip the missed dose and continue with your regular schedule.

SIDE EFFECTS: Common side effects include restlessness; insomnia; dizziness; tremors; palpitations; blurred vision; constipation; dry mouth; and change in sex drive. Uncommon effects include very high blood pressure; hallucinations; cardiac arrest; coma; convulsions; and death. On February 13, 1998, a "black box" warning was added to the product's labeling indicating that there is a risk of valvular disease and primary pulmonary hypertension when taking this drug. This type of warning is the strongest the industry issues for drugs and should be seriously considered before taking phendimetrazine.

PRECAUTIONS: Use of phendimetrazine may decrease the effectiveness of any blood pressure medications you are taking. If you use this drug along with MAO inhibitors or the antimicrobial drug furazolidone, it can raise blood pressure and your risk of stroke. If you suddenly stop taking phendimetrazine, you may experience withdrawal symptoms such as extreme fatigue, depression, and trouble sleeping.

Do not take phendimetrazine if you are pregnant, may be pregnant, or are breast-feeding. Phendimetrazine is a schedule II drug, which means it has a high potential for abuse, greater than that of other nonamphetamine stimulants.

Consult your doctor before taking phendimetrazine if you are taking any of the following drugs, as negative interactions may occur: MAO inhibitors; phenothiazine tranquilizers; antihypertensive medications; insulin or oral diabetic medications; over-the-counter cough, cold, and asthma drugs. Avoid caffeine products while taking phendimetrazine.

Phendimetrazine, like other appetite suppressants, often causes dry mouth, which can increase the chance of developing gum disease and dental cavities. Special attention to oral hygiene, including use of sugarless gum and sugarless hard candies, drinking lots of water, or sucking on ice chips, is recommended while taking these drugs.

FURTHER INFORMATION: **Print:** Hadler, A. J., Sustained-action phendimetrazine in obesity. *J Clin Pharmacol J New Drugs*, Mar.–Apr. 1968, 8(2): 113–17; Hood, I. et al., Fatality from illicit phendimetrazine use. *J Toxicol Clin Toxicol*, 1988, 26(3–4): 249–55; Rostagno, C. et al., Dilated cardiomyopathy associated with chronic consumption of phendimetrazine. *Am Heart J*, Feb. 1996, 131(2): 407–9.

Sibutramine hydrochloride monohydrate

BRAND NAME(S): Meridia; no generic available.
TYPE/DEFINITION: Sibutramine is a monoamine reuptake inhibitor and an appetite suppressant. Sibutramine was developed in the late 1980s as an antidepressant, and it was approved in

November 1997 (final approval, February 1998) by the FDA as a weight-management medication. It is a schedule IV controlled substance, with low potential for abuse.

HOW SOLD: Available in 5-, 10-, and 15-mg capsules.

RESEARCH: Researchers at Nova Southeastern University in Ft. Lauderdale, Florida (1999), conducted a double-blind, controlled study and found sibutramine to be effective in reducing weight when it is used along with a reduced-calorie diet, behavior modification, and an exercise program. They also warned that some patients experience a substantial increase in heart rate and blood pressure.

The manufacturer reports that weight loss was examined in eleven double-blind, placebo-controlled obesity trials that lasted from 12 to 52 weeks and used doses ranging from 1 to 30 mg 1 time daily. Compared with patients who took placebos, those who took 5 to 20 mg of sibutramine daily lost significantly more weight. Analysis of data from three studies that lasted 6 months or longer indicates that patients who lose at least 4 pounds during the first 4 weeks of treatment on a given dose will most likely achieve significant long-term weight loss on that same dose.

PRODUCT CLAIMS: Sibutramine is a monoamine reuptake inhibitor, which means it blocks the reabsorption of the neurotransmitters (messengers) serotonin and norepinephrine, and to a lesser extent dopamine, by the neurons that originally released them. This allows the levels of these neurotransmitters to increase, which in turn helps control appetite. Sibutramine may also assist with weight loss in other ways, but they have not yet been found. The hypothesis that sibutramine raises the metabolic rate and thus helps burn more calories was dismissed by researchers in a study published in *Obesity Research* in 1998 (see Further Information).

Studies show that after 12 months, obese individuals who took sibutramine (15 mg daily) lost an average of 10 pounds more than people who had taken a placebo. To be effective, sibutramine must be used along with a sensible eating plan, behavior modification, and a regular exercise program. However, weight loss may be temporary only, especially after the drug is discontinued. To maintain weight loss or to continue to lose additional weight after stopping sibutramine, it is necessary to follow a sensible eating plan and an exercise program.

DOSAGE INFORMATION: The recommended daily dose is 10 mg 1 time a day with or without food. If there is inadequate weight loss after 4 weeks, your physician may increase your dosage to 15 mg 1 time a day, or treatment may be discontinued. Total daily intake should not exceed 15 mg. In most of the clinical trials, the dose was taken in the morning.

Knoll Pharmaceuticals, the maker of Meridia, developed a Point of Change (SM) weight-management program to accompany the drug. This support program details lifestyle changes that you can use to create a plan that meets your specific needs. Point of Change teaches Meridia users how to record their nutrition and exercise habits, set realistic goals, and use self-assessment tools.

SIDE EFFECTS: The most common side effects are dry mouth; anorexia; headache; insomnia; and constipation. Some users experience an increase in blood pressure and heart rate.

PRECAUTIONS: If you have cardiovascular disease or high blood pressure, consult your doctor before using this drug. However, tests on humans do not show evidence of valvular heart disease when taking this drug. *Do not take sibutramine with any other appetite suppressant.* Regular medical followup is recommended while you take this drug.

Sibutramine, like other appetite suppressants, often causes dry mouth, which can increase the chance of developing gum disease and dental cavities. Special attention to oral hygiene, including use of sugarless gum and sugarless hard candies, drinking lots of water, or sucking on ice chips, is recommended while taking this drug.

FURTHER INFORMATION: **Print:** Connoley, I. P., et al., Thermogenic effects of sibutramine and its metabolites. *Br J Pharmacol*, Mar. 1999, 126(6): 1487–95; Heal, D. J., et al., Sibutramine: a novel anti-obesity drug. A review of the pharmacological evidence to differentiate it from d-amphetamine and d-fenfluramine. *Int J Obes*

Relat Metab Disord, Aug. 1998, 22 (Suppl 1): S18–28; Luque, C. A., and Rey, J. A., Sibutramine: A serotonin-norepinephrine re-uptake inhibitor for the treatment of obesity. *Anni Pharmacother*, Sep. 1999, 33(9): 968–78; Seagle, H. M., et al. *Obesity Research*, Mar. 1998, 6(2): 115–121. **Web sites:** www.rxlist.com/cgi/weight/sibutramine.htm; www.4meridia.com; www.obesity-news.com/merhirs.htm.

PART II

Single-Ingredient, Over-the-Counter
Weight-Management Products

SAY IT'S the middle of March and you're already thinking about summer and the beach . . . and the 15 pounds you've put on since last summer. Perhaps you just received an invitation to your twenty-fifth class reunion and you're thinking, "I've got three months to lose the extra 10 pounds I've gained over the past year." Is it time to run to your doctor for a diet-pill prescription?

Unless you're obese and need to lose a significant amount of weight, the answer is *no*: prescription diet pills are not for you. Although some doctors do prescribe them for people who are not obese, it is not accepted medical practice, and you may need over-the-counter (OTC) products if you want a dietary aid to help you lose 5, 10, or 20 pounds, along with a reduced-calorie eating plan and exercise program.

Over-the-counter weight-loss products have some advantages over prescription diet drugs.

- You don't need to go to your doctor for a prescription (although it is recommended that you consult with your doctor before taking any weight-loss product).
- OTC products don't have the potential for addiction as do most prescription diet drugs.
- In most cases, you can stop taking an OTC diet product without worrying about withdrawal side effects.
- Most OTC products are less expensive than prescription drugs.

HOW TO CHOOSE AN OTC DIET PRODUCT

There are dozens of OTC weight-loss products available on the market as single supplements—herbs, vitamins, minerals, other nutrients, and various other natural substances. How do you know which ones are safe and effective? To help you make an informed decision about OTC diet products, you need to have easy access to the latest information on them. That's what you'll find in this part.

To help you evaluate the merits of each ingredient, Part II offers you information about the research (if any), both positive and negative, that has been done on each substance; the dosages reported to cause weight loss; dosage information, including a list of medicines and other items that may interact with it; side effects and precautions; and where to look for further, in-depth information. When little or no research has been done or published, anecdotal information is included. In some cases, anecdotal reports are the only evidence available for the claims made about a substance.

The information in this section can benefit you in two ways. First, it can help you decide whether a particular single substance is an effective and safe weight-loss product. Second, if you are considering a combination weight-loss product (see Part III), you can learn about each individual ingredient in the combination product to see whether that product contains substances that are safe and that are present in amounts sufficient to promote weight loss. Although not every ingredient you may find in a combination product is described, it does include those that are most commonly found in such items. For brief explanations of less commonly used ingredients, as well as fillers that are used in the manufacture of tablets and capsules, see the Glossary (pp. 183–90). There you will find a brief description of these ingredients as they relate to weight loss.

Every effort has been made to provide the latest information on the substances included in this part. However, new studies and findings become available from time to time, and they may alter the information presented here. Also, manufacturers change formulas, drop products from their line, add new ones, and sometimes simply make a name change. Be an informed consumer. Let these pages be your guide, but also be alert to new findings as they become available.

DIET TERMS YOU'LL SEE IN PART II

Here are a few terms you'll see in the following entries.

- Appetite suppressant: a substance that reduces hunger and the desire to eat.
- Diuretic: a substance that increases the flow of urine from the body.
- Laxative: a substance that loosens the bowels and causes them to eliminate their contents. Some laxatives work by softening the bowel contents; others increase the bulk of the contents.
- Thermogenic agent: a substance that promotes the transformation of calories into heat ("burning calories").

BEST BETS

These substances have been selected as "best bets" for weight-loss aids because some scientific studies have shown them to be safe and effective in human studies. They may facilitate weight loss if used with a reduced-calorie diet and an exercise program. Other weight-loss aids also appear to be safe and effective, but these qualities have not been proven in reliable scientific studies.

Glucomannan: This substance provides a feeling of satiety, thus suppressing your appetite.

Green tea: Scientific research shows that green tea boosts metabolism, and it has the added benefits of being an antioxidant and a possible cancer-preventive substance.

BEST BETS (*Cont.*)

Guar gum: This substance provides a feeling of satiety, thus suppressing your appetite.

5-HTP: This amino acid suppresses carbohydrate cravings.

Psyllium: This substance provides a feeling of satiety, thus suppressing your appetite.

Carnitine (L-carnitine)

MANUFACTURERS/BRAND NAME(S): Doctor's A-Z, Twinlab, Natrol, among others.

HOW SOLD: Capsules, 250 mg and 500 mg; tablets, 500 mg. Carnitine comes in three forms: L- , D- , and DL-carnitine. The form associated with weight management is L-carnitine.

TYPE/DEFINITION: In regard to weight loss, L-carnitine is a thermogenic agent. Generally, it is a nonessential (which means the body can produce it) amino acid that is manufactured in the liver and kidneys, where it is converted from two other nonessential amino acids, lysine and methionine. It is sometimes referred to as a "vitamin-like" compound because it is a popular nutritional supplement used to help remove fat from the blood.

BACKGROUND/RESEARCH: Studies show that people who are overweight or obese often have immune systems that are less able to destroy bacteria, which causes them to get more infections than normal-weight individuals. Overweight people also tend to have elevated levels of cholesterol and other fatty substances (lipids) in their bloodstream, which are believed to be associated with their impaired immune function.

Several studies suggest that L-carnitine helps overcome the negative effects that high levels of cholesterol and lipids have on the immune system in people who are overweight or obese. This may be due to the ability of L-carnitine to remove fats from the blood. It also has been suggested that the ability of L-carnitine to help build muscle, which in turn uses energy and burns fat, may promote weight loss.

But a recent study casts doubt on that idea. In a double-blind, placebo-controlled study, researchers in Australia gave L-carnitine to thirteen overweight premenopausal women and placebo to fifteen. For 8 weeks, both groups of women got the same diet and amount of physical exercise, and at the end of the study, there was no significant difference in the changes in total body mass or fat mass. Therefore, the researchers concluded that their results cast "doubt on the efficacy of L-carnitine supplementation for weight loss." The scientists also noted that five of the women who were taking L-carnitine eventually dropped out of the study because of nausea and diarrhea attributed to the L-carnitine.

PRODUCT CLAIMS: L-carnitine plays a significant part in the metabolism of fat and may reduce feelings of hunger. It helps transport fat into the mitochondria, which is the energy center in a cell. During weight-loss programs, as the body eliminates (burns) stored fats, it produces ketones. If L-carnitine levels are low, the body is unable to transport the fats into the mitochondria for breakdown. Taking supplements of L-carnitine could help the body rid itself of the excess fats. L-carnitine also helps keep energy levels up, because the mitochondria use the fats to produce fuel for the body. However, there is no convincing evidence that carnitine deficiency is common in the United States or that supplemental carnitine does promote weight loss.

DOSAGE INFORMATION: To effectively metabolize fats, carnitine needs adequate levels of vitamin C. A typical dosage of carnitine is 1,500 to 4,000 mg per day, which should be taken along with 500 to 1,000 mg vitamin C, which requires supplements as a typical diet provides less than 100 mg daily.

Some experts believe that the potential for abuse when taking amino acids is too great and that their use should be discouraged. Therefore, consult your physician before taking this supplement. Generally, health-care providers agree that taking a single amino acid can create an imbalance of the other amino-acid levels in the body.

SIDE EFFECTS: The most common side effects are body odor and gastrointestinal disorders, such as nausea, diarrhea, and stomach

pain. There is a slight risk of kidney problems with L-carnitine.
PRECAUTIONS: *Do not take DL-carnitine.* Even though it has
some of the properties of L-carnitine, it can cause debilitating
muscle weakness.
FURTHER INFORMATION: **Print:** Simone, D. et al. "Vitamins and
immunity II: Influence of L-carnitine on the immune system.
Acta Vit Enz, 1982, 4:135–40; Simone, D. et al., Reversibility
by L-carnitine of immunosuppression induced by an emulsion
of soya bean oil, glycerol, and egg lecithin." *Arzneim Forsch,*
1982, 32: 1488; Villani, R. G., et al., L-carnitine supplementation combined with aerobic training does not promote weight
loss in moderately obese women. *Int Sport Nut,* June 2000,
10(2):199–207. Also see Crayhon, Robert, *The Carnitine Miracle: The Supernutrient Program That Promotes High Energy,
Fat Burning, Heart Health, Brain Wellness and Longevity,* M.
Evans & Co., 1998; Schwartz, Erika, M.D., *Natural Energy:
From Tired to Terrific in 10 Days,* Putnam, 1999.

Cascara sagrada (*Rhamnus purshiana cortex*)
(also known as buckthorn)

MANUFACTURERS/BRAND NAME(S): Frontier, Herb Pharm, Nature's Way, Nature's Herbs, Gaia Herbs, Enrich Corporation,
Nature's Sunshine, among others.
HOW SOLD: Capsules (usually 400 mg), tablets, tincture, extract, dried bark.
TYPE/DEFINITION: Stimulant/laxative. Cascara sagrada is obtained from the bark and black berries of the buckthorn tree,
which is native to the mountainous areas of North America.
BACKGROUND/RESEARCH: The use of this plant as a laxative and
stimulant is primarily anecdotal and steeped in centuries' old
tradition. No controlled scientific studies have been published.
Use of cascara sagrada as a dietary aid is not recommended.
PRODUCT CLAIMS: Cascara stimulates contractions of the large
intestine, which encourages elimination. The main compounds
responsible for this action are chemicals called anthraquinones,
which make up 6 to 9 percent of the bark. Cascara also causes

fluid loss, so you can expect a temporary, limited amount of weight reduction due to water loss. However, cascara does not promote fat loss and therefore is not recommended for weight loss.

DOSAGE INFORMATION: Although many people take cascara sagrada to help them lose weight, experts strongly discourage this use of the herb. Cascara sagrada should be used only to relieve severe constipation. For that purpose, it can be taken either with or without food. A typical dosage is 40 to 60 drops of tincture or extract in water in the morning and evening. The dried form (1 to 2 teaspoons) can be added to 8 ounces of boiling water and allowed to steep for 10 minutes. Package directions typically suggest drinking 1 to 2 cups per day on an empty stomach. The manufacturer suggests taking 1 to 2 capsules or tablets per day. Always take cascara with water.

SIDE EFFECTS: Cascara sagrada can cause diarrhea; discolored urine (yellow-brown to red); vomiting; dehydration; electrolyte imbalance; and stomach or intestinal cramps.

PRECAUTIONS: Herbalists warn that cascara is a very powerful laxative and should only be used as a last resort for severe cases of constipation. Cascara should never be used with any other laxative. Do not take if you are pregnant or breast-feeding, as it can pass into the breast milk. Avoid cascara if you have Crohn's disease; ulcerative colitis; appendicitis; unexplained abdominal pain; or if you are taking any of the following medications: cardiac glycosides; antiarrhythmics; thiazide diuretics; licorice; or corticosteroids. Use of cascara with a diuretic such as uva ursi or caffeine can cause dehydration and a loss of electrolytes (potassium, magnesium, and calcium). If this mineral imbalance is not corrected, it can cause muscle weakness and dangerous disturbances of heart rhythm.

Do not use cascara sagrada for longer than 8 to 10 days without first consulting your doctor. Prolonged use (2 weeks or more) can cause lazy bowel syndrome, which means stool will not move through the intestines without chemical stimulation. In other words, it can become habit-forming.

When purchasing cascara sagrada, look for products that say the bark was aged for at least 1 year or was artificially treated with heat and aeration before it was packaged. Bark that has been incorrectly harvested or processed can cause severe cramping and vomiting. *Never use fresh cascara.*

FURTHER INFORMATION: **Print:** Editors, *Drug & Natural Medicine Advisor: The Complete Guide to Alternative & Conventional Medications*, Time/Life, 1997. **Contact/Web site:** American Botanical Council, PO Box 201660, Austin TX 78720; 1-800-373-7105; www.herbalgram.org.

Cayenne (*Capsicum frutescens*)

MANUFACTURERS/BRAND NAME(S): Nature's Way, Nature's Herbs, among others.

HOW SOLD: Capsules, usually 400 to 500 mg; or 100,000 IU (international units); also powder.

TYPE/DEFINITION: Thermogenic agent. Cayenne is a plant native to tropical America, but now it is widely cultivated. It is also known as American pepper, chili pepper, red pepper, and Spanish pepper. Herbalists consider cayenne to be a powerful tonic that has an overall invigorating effect on the body.

BACKGROUND/RESEARCH: Most of the evidence that cayenne is useful for weight loss is anecdotal. However, researchers at a laboratory in Quebec, Canada, report that capsaicin (the active ingredient in cayenne pepper) has the ability to increase metabolism. At the Oxford Polytechnic Institute in England, scientists observed that the metabolic rate increased as much as 25 percent in subjects who included 1 teaspoon red pepper sauce and 1 teaspoon mustard with their meals.

PRODUCT CLAIMS: Capsaicin promotes blood flow and perspiration, which helps rid the body of wastes. It also speeds up the metabolism. Cayenne (capsaicin) is often found in combination weight-loss products that contain other thermogenic substances (e.g., guarana, garcinia cambogia), because it stimulates their actions. Ironically, cayenne is also used to stimulate the appetite.

DOSAGE INFORMATION: If you use the cayenne powder, experts suggest you start with about ⅛ teaspoon mixed into your food at each meal. Gradually increase the amount to ¼ teaspoon at each meal. To take an infusion, experts suggest pouring 8 ounces boiling water onto ½ to 1 teaspoon cayenne powder and allowing it to steep for 10 minutes. Then they recommend adding 1 teaspoon of the infusion to several ounces of hot water. Always take cayenne with food to prevent irritation of the stomach lining.

SIDE EFFECTS: When used as directed, there are usually no side effects, apart from the familiar hot sensation in the mouth, and sometimes the anus during a bowel movement after taking a large dose of cayenne. In rare cases or when taken in large doses, it may cause diarrhea, nausea, or vomiting. Contrary to popular opinion, cayenne does not cause ulcers; in fact, it is used to improve digestion and relieve gas.

PRECAUTIONS: If cayenne is taken in excess of the recommended amounts, it can cause kidney or liver damage and gastroenteritis. If you have gastritis, bowel disease, or ulcers, consult your physician before taking cayenne.

FURTHER INFORMATION: **Print:** Doucet E., and Tremblay, A., Food intake, energy balance and body weight control. *Eur J Clin Nutr*, Dec. 1997, 51 (12): 846–55; Editors, *Drug & Natural Medicine Advisor: The Complete Guide to Alternative & Conventional Medications,* Time/Life 1997; Quillin, Patrick, *Healing Power of Cayenne Pepper: Complete Handbook of Cayenne Home Remedies,* Leader Co. Inc., 1999. **Contact/ Web site:** American Botanical Council, PO Box 201660, Austin TX 78720; 1-800-373-7105; www.herbalgram.org.

Chickweed (*Stelleria media*)

MANUFACTURERS/BRAND NAMES(S): Nature's Herbs, Frontier, Nature's Answer, Nature's Way, Gaia Herbs, among others.

HOW SOLD: Dried bulk tea, capsules, tincture.

TYPE/DEFINITION: Chickweed is a diuretic, laxative, and appetite suppressant. The plant is widely regarded as a bothersome weed and can be found growing around the world. It is also known as Adder's mouth, satin flower, and starwort.

BACKGROUND/RESEARCH: Only anecdotal evidence is available to support claims that chickweed is effective for weight loss, yet it is commonly used in dietary products. It is also high in vitamin C, and it can be eaten raw or cooked, as you would spinach. Components in chickweed called saponin glycosides give this herb soothing qualities for both internal use and topical use for skin problems.

PRODUCT CLAIMS: Chickweed is rich in lecithin, a natural substance found in the cell membranes. Lecithin is a fat emulsifier, which means it dissolves fats in watery fluids such as blood serum. It is claimed that this allows the body to process and transport body fat and thus aid in weight loss, although scientific proof of this process is lacking.

DOSAGE INFORMATION: To make an infusion, experts recommend pouring 16 ounces of boiling water over 1 ounce of dried chickweed and steeping for 15 minutes. The suggested dose is 3 or more cups daily. For the tincture, the recommended dose is up to 60 drops in water daily. Chickweed can also be eaten raw in salads or cooked, like spinach. It is a rich source of vitamin C.

SIDE EFFECTS: No side effects are expected when using this herb.

PRECAUTIONS: No precautions are associated with this herb.

FURTHER INFORMATION: **Print:** Editors, *Drug & Natural Medicine Advisor: The Complete Guide to Alternative & Conventional Medications*, Time/Life, 1997. **Contact/Web site:** American Botanical Council, PO Box 201660, Austin TX 78720; 1-800-373-7105; www.herbalgram.org

Chitin, chitosan (a processed version of chitin)

MANUFACTURERS/BRAND NAME(S): Fat Absorb™, Chitosorb, Chinese HD, and Discover, among others.

HOW SOLD: Tablets and capsules, typically 500 mg.

TYPE/DEFINITION: Fat absorber. Chitin is a fiber product derived from the exoskeletons of marine animals, such as crabs, oysters, and other shellfish, or from the exoskeletons of some insects. It was originally used in industrial settings to soak up oil, grease, and other toxic substances from liquid, including drinking water.

BACKGROUND/RESEARCH: Chitosan has a mixed reputation. Some experts hail it as an important weight-loss substance because of its ability to collect and eliminate fatty deposits in the intestines. Some advocates of the product say it can promote blood clotting, treat ulcers, prevent tooth decay, and treat staph infections.

Not everyone is convinced of chitosan's virtues. In March 2001, researchers at the University of California at Davis Clinical Nutrition Research Unit found that chitosan does not block the absorption of fat. Nor is the Federal Trade Commission convinced. In 1999, the commission charged one manufacturer of chitosan with false advertising and failure to prove the claims they were making. Those claims include the ability to promote weight loss, lower the risk of cancer, reduce cholesterol levels, control blood pressure, and heal infections. (See **Enforma System,** Part III, pp. 129–30.) Another question about chitin is its purity and composition, which can vary greatly depending on which animal it is extracted from, where it is harvested, and the time of year it is gathered.

Up until 1999, no scientific studies had been conducted on the use of chitin in humans. Claims of weight loss were based on studies done in mice, in which chitin lowered blood-sugar, cholesterol, and triglyceride levels in normal-weight animals. It had no effect on obese mice. When chitin was added to chicken feed, the chickens that ate the treated food were leaner than those that ate untreated feed. Then, in 1999, the results of a placebo-controlled, double-blind trial showed that chitosan, when taken by overweight individuals who did not change their diet, did not result in weight loss.

Gary Huber, vice president for Scientific Affairs in the American Nutraceutical Association in Birmingham, Alabama, says that even in the studies that involved chickens and other animals, the amount of chitin given during the experiments was "huge." "[Humans] would have to take several cupfuls," he says, in order to notice any benefit from chitin. However, even much smaller amounts of chitin can cause problems (see Precautions).

PRODUCT CLAIMS: Chitin has no calories because it is not digestible. Claims by manufacturers of chitosan products are that it binds to or captures excess fat molecules and can reduce fat absorption by 20 to 30 percent. Chitosan reportedly absorbs 6 to 8 times its weight in fats and oils, as well as controls blood pressure, has antitumor action, increases bone density, heals wounds, lowers LDL (low-density lipoprotein, the "bad" cholesterol) by as much as 66 percent, and increases HDL (high-density lipoprotein, the "good" cholesterol). Many experts agree that these claims are greatly exaggerated. According to David Schardt, associate nutritionist for the Center for Science in the Public Interest, "it's conceivable that it may have a small effect," but that effect is almost unnoticeable.

DOSAGE INFORMATION: A typical dosage is at least 1 gram 30 minutes before or with lunch or dinner. Drink at least 8 ounces of water with each tablet to help prevent constipation, and drink at least an additional 48 ounces of water throughout the day.

SIDE EFFECTS: Many packages say no side effects have been reported when it is taken as directed. However, anecdotal reports tell of the potential for diarrhea and fatty stools.

PRECAUTIONS: Chitosan interferes with the absorption of fat-soluble vitamins (vitamins A, D, and E) and fat-soluble drugs. A deficiency of these vitamins can occur when taking chitosan. Never take more than 3 grams of chitosan a day, or severe constipation may occur. *If you are allergic to shellfish, do not take chitosan.* Chitosan will not promote weight loss in individuals who binge and purge or who regularly overeat. Children younger than fourteen should not take chitosan. Do not take it if you are pregnant or breast-feeding. Because fiber supplements can interfere with the effectiveness and action of prescription and nonprescription drugs, nutritional supplements, and herbal remedies, consult your doctor before taking chitosan if you are taking any of these substances.

FURTHER INFORMATION: **Print:** Deuchi, K. et al., Decreasing effect of chitosan on the apparent fat digestibility by rats fed on a high-fat diet. *Biosc Biotech Biochem* 1994, 58: 1613–16; Nauss, J. L. et al., The binding of micellar lipids to chitosan. *Lipids*, 1995, 18 (10): 714–19; Pitfler. M. H., et al., Randomized, double-blind trial of chitosan for body weight reduction. *Eur J Clin Nut*, May 1999, 53 (5): 379–81. Also see Henneni, William, *Chitosan*, Woodland, 1996; Simontacchi Carol, *All About Chitosan*, Avery, 1999.

Chromium picolinate

MANUFACTURERS/BRAND NAME(S): Schiff, Nature Made, Solgar, Twinlab, among others.

HOW SOLD: Tablets, capsules, usually 100 and 200 mg.

TYPE/DEFINITION: Thermogenic agent. Chromium is an essential mineral found naturally in the body and in some foods, such as apples, broccoli, green peppers, mushrooms, potatoes, and brewer's yeast. Although no Recommended Daily Allowance (RDA) has been set for chromium, the EMDR (estimated mimimum daily requirement) is 50 mcg to 200 mcg. Chromium alone is not well absorbed by the body, which is why it is commonly chelated (bound) to other substances, such as picolinate.

BACKGROUND/RESEARCH: The claim that chromium picolinate can enhance metabolic rate was initiated by Gary Evans, Ph.D., a chemist at Bemidji State University in Minnesota. Dr. Evans conducted a study in which forty-one athletes were given either 200 mcg of chromium or a placebo. The athletes who took the chromium had reduced body fat and increased muscle mass. This study formed the basis for subsequent claims that the mineral was an effective supplement for weight loss.

Some researchers dispute the health and weight-loss claims attributed to chromium picolinate. Among them are Ellen Coleman, R.D., M.A., M.P.H., who wrote in The Chromium Picolinate Weight Loss Scam, *Sports Medicine Digest*, 1997, 19 (1):6–7, that "the success of chromium picolinate is due to a remarkably well-orchestrated marketing campaign initiated by both Nutrition 21 (a San Diego, California–based food-supplement company) and their consultant chemist, Gary Evans (who also authored *Chromium Picolinate*)." Nutrition 21 holds the exclusive U.S. license to the patent rights to the supplement. Picolinic acid is believed to facilitate the absorption of chromium. According to Ms. Coleman, studies conducted by Dr. Evans, who once worked for the USDA on the synthesis of picolinates and then joined Bemidji State University, where he researched and promoted chromium picolinate as a weight-loss product, were poorly controlled and contain unsubstantiated information.

Several studies support Ms. Coleman's claims that chromium picolinate is not effective in reducing weight, increasing muscular strength, or improving muscle mass. In 1995, a study published by the *Journal of Sports Medicine and Physical Fitness* involved ninety-five overweight, active-duty Navy personnel who were given 400 mcg chromium picolinate or placebo while engaged in an exercise program. After 16 weeks, both groups had lost a similar amount of weight and body fat and had a similar increase in lean body mass. "It was concluded that chromium picolinate was ineffective in enhancing body-fat reduction in this group and could not be recommended as an adjuvant to Navy weight-loss programs in general."

In 1996, researchers at the USDA Human Nutrition Research Center in Beltsville, Maryland, studied the effects of chromium picolinate or placebo on subjects who were started on a weight-lifting program. After 3 months, subjects in both groups had similar changes in strength and body composition. Another study, conducted by Henry Lukaski, Ph.D., and his colleagues at the USDA that same year, had similar results. Thus in November 1996, the Federal Trade Commission ordered all companies that made and distributed chromium picolinate to stop claiming that it was an effective weight-loss agent until they could support those statements with reliable research.

There is also evidence that chromium may be harmful. Several studies (see Side Effects) show that chromium is retained in the cells, where it places oxidative stress on the DNA and may promote cancer.

Chromium picolinate is not the only type of chromium you will see in weight-loss products on the market, so a few words about the other types need to be said. The term *chromium GTF* refers to glucose tolerance factor, which is the term given to this form of chromium when it was first discovered that chromium had an effect on blood-sugar levels. A form of chromium GTF is chromium polynicotinate, which is commonly used but not as well absorbed as chromium picolinate. According to the Chromium Information Bureau, it is not really known why chromium picolinate is better absorbed than other chromium forms. Other forms of chromium include those that have been chelated with one or more amino acids, such as chromium chelate and chromium chelavite. These amino-acid chromium chelates are not as well studied in humans as they have been in animals. (For more information about chromium, see Further Information.)

PRODUCT CLAIMS: When the body digests carbohydrates, it releases a hormone called insulin, which is involved in the production of energy and in keeping body fat low and lean muscle high. Chromium is a cofactor, or helper, to insulin, and so it helps increase insulin's ability to reduce the amount of body fat. Insulin helps reduce body fat because it plays a key role in fat metabolism. Some researchers suggest that chromium can reduce the carbohydrate cravings often associated with type II diabetes or insulin resistance, and in this way contributes to weight loss. However, benefit is only likely to occur in people who have a chromium deficiency, which is not a common problem in the generally well-fed U.S. population.

DOSAGE INFORMATION: The manufacturers' suggested amount of chromium picolinate to take for weight loss is 200 to 400 mcg per day for women and 400 to 600 mcg per day for men. The doses can be taken 2 times a day and should be taken with food.

SIDE EFFECTS: There have been rare reports of irregular heartbeat when chromium is taken at high doses.

Following a 1995 study conducted by the George Washington University Department of Pharmacology (Chromium Toxicity Study) in which investigators found that chromium picolinate caused chromosomal damage in cultured hamster cancer cells, the USDA Human Nutrition Research Center conducted its own review. The USDA reported that no harmful effects could be attributed to chromium picolinate when it was given to animals.

PRECAUTIONS: Some research shows that dosages of 1,000 mcg or more taken over weeks or months may be toxic to the liver and kidneys and may disrupt the ability of insulin to perform properly.

FURTHER INFORMATION: **Print:** Dubrovskaya, V. A., and Wetterhahn, K. E., Effects of Cr(VI) on the expression of the oxidative stress genes in human lung cells. *Carcinogenesis*, Aug. 1998, 19(8): 1401–7; Evans, G. W., The effect of chromium picolinate on insulin-controlled parameters in humans. *Int J Biosoc Med and Res,* 1989, 11: 163–180; Hallmark, M. A., et al., Effects of chromium and resistive training on muscle strength and body composition. *Med and Sci in Sports and Exercise*, 1996, 28: 139–44; Lukaski, H. C., et al., Chromium supplementation and resistance training: effects on body composition, strength, and trace element status of men. *Amer J Clin Nut*, 1996, 63: 954–65; Trent, L. K., and Thieding-Cancel, D., Effects of chromium picolinate on body composition. *J Sports Med Phys Fitness*, Dec. 1995, 35(4):273–80. **Contact/Web site:** Chromium Information Bureau, a nonprofit educational organization, at www.chromiuminfo.org.

Citrus aurantium (in Chinese medicine, zhi shi)

MANUFACTURERS/BRAND NAME(S): Natrol, among others.

TYPE/DEFINITION: Thermogenic agent. Citrus aurantium is derived from the citrus rinds of the bitter orange while the fruit is still green.

HOW SOLD: Capsules, typically 250 mg.

BACKGROUND/RESEARCH: Citrus aurantium has long been used in traditional Chinese medicine to treat indigestion and to promote circulation and liver health. Much of the evidence about the weight-loss ability of citrus aurantium is anecdotal and has been passed down from generation to generation in various cultures. A scientific study conducted in 1999 looked at the anti-obesity effects of an extract of citrus aurantium in rats. The researchers did find that the extract "significantly reduced food intake and body weight gain" in the rats. Studies in people, however, are lacking.

PRODUCT CLAIMS: Citrus aurantium is a rich source of flavonoids, vitamins A, B, and C, and several alkaloids that have the ability to break down fat and raise resting metabolism levels. Two of these alkaloids are synephrine and nobiletin. Small amounts of synephrine can increase energy and improve digestion, and nobiletin protects against some cancers and regulates secretions in the intestinal tract. A combination of citrus aurantium and moderate physical activity is reported to be very effective in weight loss.

DOSAGE INFORMATION: A typical dosage of citrus aurantium is generally 1 capsule per day, with food.

SIDE EFFECTS: Citrus aurantium has no known side effects, although studies are limited. Unlike some other thermogenic substances, such as ephedra (ephedrine), citrus aurantium supposedly does not increase heart rate or blood pressure or cause agitation.

PRECAUTIONS: Although no studies have shown it to be harmful to pregnant or breast-feeding women, it is best to avoid this supplement during pregnancy and lactation.

FURTHER INFORMATION: **Print:** Calapai, G., et al., Antiobesity and cardiovascular toxic effects of citrus aurantium extracts in the rat: a preliminary report. *Fitoterapia*, 1999, 70(6): 586–92; Colker, C. M., et al., Effects of citrus aurantium extract, caffeine, and St. John's wort on body fat loss, lipid levels, and mood states in overweight healthy adults. *Curr Ther Res*, 1999, 60: 145–53.

Coenzyme Q10

MANUFACTURERS/BRAND NAME(S): Natrol, Carlson Labs, Schiff, Twinlab, Futurebiotics, among others.

TYPE/DEFINITION: Thermogenic agent. Coenzyme Q10 (or ubiquinone) is a fat-soluble substance manufactured by the body and a powerful antioxidant. It is found in cells throughout the body.

HOW SOLD: Capsules, softgels, chewable wafers, sublingual lozenges, 20 to 100 mg.

BACKGROUND/RESEARCH: Levels of Co Q10 decline as people age, and this fact has led many experts to believe that supplementation may slow down the aging process. Therefore, much research has focused on the impact of Co Q10 supplementation on reducing the risk of heart attack, lowering blood pressure, boosting the immune system, slowing Alzheimer's disease, and other aspects of aging.

Very little research has been done on the use of Co Q10 for weight loss, although a substantial amount has been done in regard to its benefits in heart disease, periodontal disease, hypertension, and diabetes. An exploratory study done in the 1980s found that individuals who had a family history of obesity had a 50 percent reduced ability to burn calories after eating a meal and also had low Co Q10 levels. This led the scientists to suggest that supplementing with the enzyme could help with weight loss.

One physician who believes there is a connection between Co Q10 and obesity is Melvyn Werbach, M.D., author of *Healing with Food*. Another is Julian Whitaker, M.D., author of *Dr. Whitaker's Guide to Natural Healing*, who believes that low levels of Co Q10 may be a significant factor in poor thermogenesis in people who are obese.

PRODUCT CLAIMS: Some experts recommend supplementation with Co Q10 for overweight people because they believe it speeds up fat metabolism, and some overweight individuals have low levels of the enzyme. However, it is unknown what proportion of overweight individuals have low levels of coenzyme Q10 or how effective it may be for weight loss.

DOSAGE INFORMATION: Dr. Whitaker recommends taking 20 to 30 mg Co Q10 3 times daily, while Dr. Werbach suggests a similar amount: 50 mg 2 times daily. Always take Co Q10 with food. For maximum absorption and effectiveness, take it with food that contains some fat, such as almonds, peanut butter, or vegetables served with olive oil. It is also important to consume enough vitamin E when taking Co Q10, because vitamin E stimulates the natural production of the enzyme. Take 400 to 800 IU vitamin E daily. If you are taking blood thinners, consult your doctor before taking vitamin E.

SIDE EFFECTS: No side effects have been reported.

PRECAUTIONS: Do not take Co Q10 if you are pregnant or breast-feeding. If you have heart disease, consult your doctor before taking this supplement.

FURTHER INFORMATION: **Print:** van Gaal, L., de Leeuw, I. D., Vadhanavikit, S., and Folkers, K., Exploratory study of coenzyme Q10 in obesity. In Folkers, K., and Yamamura, Y. (eds.)., *Biomedical and Clinical Aspects of Coenzyme Q10*, vol. 4, Elsevier, 1984, pp. 369–73. Also see Bliznakov, Emile G., *The Miracle Nutrient Coenzyme Q10*, Bantam, 1986; Murray, Michael, N.D., *Encyclopedia of Nutritional Supplements*, Prima, 1996; Sahelian, Ray, *All About Coenzyme Q10*, Avery, 1999; Sinatra, Stephen, M.D., *Coenzyme Q10 Miracle Treatment: New Hope For the Heart, Cancer, Diabetes, More*, Keats, 1998.

CLA (conjugated linoleic acid)

MANUFACTURERS/BRAND NAME(S): Twinlab, Doctor's A-Z, Wellness for Women, Natrol, among others.

TYPE/DEFINITION: Thermogenic agent. CLA is an essential fatty acid (an omega-6) that is found naturally in dairy products, beef, poultry, and corn oil.

HOW SOLD: Softgel capsules, usually 600 to 1,000 mg.

BACKGROUND/RESEARCH: Animal research suggests that CLA may reduce body fat, but so far few human studies have been done. In one of the animal studies, CLA was given to laboratory animals for 6 weeks. After 6 weeks, the CLA group had 4.3 percent body fat compared with the untreated group, which had 10.1 percent. Another animal study compared the amount of lean mass and found that CLA caused a greater growth of lean mass in animals that received CLA than in those that did not. In yet another animal study, researchers at the

University of Georgia believe their results show that the loss in fat mass caused by CLA is the result of a reduction in the size of the fat cells rather than a change in the number of fat cells.

In one of the few human studies done, researchers at the University of Wisconsin's Food Research Institute gave volunteers CLA for 3 months. The subjects lost 20 percent body fat and increased their lean muscle mass.

PRODUCT CLAIMS: Some researchers believe CLA attaches itself to the cell membrane, regulates metabolism, and breaks down the fat stored in the cells. Until further research is done, the exact mechanism of action will remain uncertain.

DOSAGE INFORMATION: Some researchers recommend taking 3 to 5g daily for weight loss. However, others believe that until adequate studies in humans have been completed, the appropriate amount to take remains unknown and so the supplement is best avoided.

SIDE EFFECTS: Because so few studies have been done in humans, the side effects are unknown. However, one unpublished human study reported a few cases of gastrointestinal disturbances.

PRECAUTIONS: CLA is believed to increase production of prostaglandins, which may increase blood circulation. Therefore, consult your physician before taking CLA if you are also taking anticoagulants.

FURTHER INFORMATION: **Print:** Azain, M. J., et al., "Dietary conjugated linoleic acid reduces rat adipose tissue cell size rather than cell number. *J Nutr*, June 2000, 130(6): 1548–54; Torkos, S., and Fitzgerald, F., *Winning at Weight Loss*. IMPAKT Communications, 1999; West, D. B., et al., Effects of conjugated linoleic acid on body fat and energy metabolism in the mouse. *Am J Physiol*, 1998, 275:R667–72; Park, Y., et al., Effect of conjugated linoleic acid on body composition in mice. *Lipids*, 1997, 32:853–58; Sugano, M., et al., Conjugated linoleic acid modulates tissue levels of chemical mediators and immunoglobulins in rats. *Lipids*, 1998, 33:521–27.

Creatine monohydrate

MANUFACTURERS/BRAND NAME(S): ProLab, ISP Powder, Ultimate Nutrition, Source Naturals, Prolab Nutrition, Twinlab, among others.

TYPE/DEFINITION: A naturally occurring chemical in the body found mainly in the liver, pancreas, and kidneys. It concentrates primarily in muscle, including the heart.

HOW SOLD: Powder, capsules, tablets, wafers, gum.

BACKGROUND/RESEARCH: Several controlled studies show that taking 20 grams per day of creatine monohydrate for 5 to 6 days can improve performance in sedentary or mildly active people when they engage in high-intensity activities such as sprinting and weight lifting. However, creatine does not seem to help endurance and also *promotes rather than hinders weight gain.*

PRODUCT CLAIMS: Studies suggest that the primary benefit of creatine supplementation is that it enhances the intensity, strength, and endurance of athletes by replacing the creatine that is used up during exercise by the muscles. Although it also helps burn fat, creatine is used primarily by athletes who want to build lean muscle mass while losing body fat; thus generally there is no net weight loss.

DOSAGE INFORMATION: Experts report the most benefit in terms of strength gains and fat loss comes when taking 5 grams 4 times a day for up to 6 days, then stopping. They also recommend taking creatine with at least 8 ounces of water, and drinking at least 64 ounces of water per day.

SIDE EFFECTS: Creatine often interferes with the body's ability to sweat, so water retention is a common problem. Unfortunately, there are no reliable studies of the long-term effects of creatine use. Anecdotal reports have associated creatine use with renal failure, muscle cramps, and muscle strains.

PRECAUTIONS: Use creatine at your own risk and only under the supervision of a doctor. Stop taking the supplement if you experience muscle cramps, muscle spasms, pulls, or strains.

FURTHER INFORMATION: **Print:** Earnest, C. P., The effect of creatine monohydrate ingestion on anaerobic power indices, muscular strength and body composition. *Acta Physciol Scand*, 1995, 207–9; Grindstaff, P. D., et al., Effects of creatine supplementation on repetitive sprint performance and body composition in competitive swimmers. *Int J Sports Nutr*, 1997, 7:330–46; Greenhaff, P. L., Creatine and its applications as an ergogenic aid. *Intl J Sport Nutr*, June 1995, 5 (Suppl):5100–10; Greenhaff, P. L., Renal dysfunction accompanying oral creatine supplements. *Lancet*, July 18, 1998, 352(9123): 233–34; Pepping, J., Creatine. *Am J Health Syst Pharm*, 1999, A9. Also see Burke, Edmund, *Creatine: What You Need to Know*, Avery, 1999; Malloy, Terry, and Monaco, Robert, *Creatine and Other Natural Muscle Boosters*, Dell, 1999.

Dandelion (*Taraxacum officinale*)

MANUFACTURERS/BRAND NAME(S): Gaia Herbs, Nature's Answer, Nature's Herbs, Nature's Way, Solaray Dandelion, Alvita (tea), among others.

HOW SOLD: Dried or fresh roots and leaves; tincture, prepared tea, capsules, powder.

TYPE/DEFINITION: An herb commonly used as a diuretic. Dandelion is rich in potassium, phosphorus, iron, and vitamin A; also a good source of calcium and vitamin B, C, and D.

BACKGROUND/RESEARCH: Evidence of dandelion's effectiveness as a weight-loss aid is largely anecdotal and has a long history. In fact, dandelion was first used as a diuretic in the tenth century by Arab physicians. Yet scientists today have not identified the exact compounds responsible for dandelion's health benefits. This fact has not stopped herbalists from recommending this herb.

PRODUCT CLAIMS: Dandelion promotes urination and the loss of water weight. Unlike many chemical diuretics, however, dandelion does not deplete the body of potassium. Dandelion also reportedly destroys the acid that builds up in overweight individuals who are on a calorie-restrictive eating plan.

DOSAGE INFORMATION: To make a decoction, experts usually suggest boiling 2 to 3 teaspoons of powdered dandelion root in

8 ounces of water for 15 minutes. If you use dried leaves, they recommend placing ½ teaspoon of leaves in 8 ounces of boiling water and allowing them to steep for 15 minutes. Package directions typically suggest drinking up to 3 cups of either preparation daily. To use the extract, manufacturers suggest adding 1 to 4 mL to water and drinking it 3 times a day. For capsules, package instructions generally suggest three 475-mg capsules 3 times daily.

SIDE EFFECTS: Dandelion is generally safe if used as directed. In rare cases it may cause stomach upset; diarrhea; rash; flulike symptoms; or liver pain.

PRECAUTIONS: Do not use dandelion if you are pregnant or breast-feeding. Before taking dandelion, consult your doctor if you have a heart condition or an inflamed colon or stomach; if you are taking potassium or lithium; or if you are taking diuretics. If you plan to take this herb for longer than 2 to 3 months, first consult your doctor. If you are older than age sixty-five, reduced doses should be taken; consult your doctor.

FURTHER INFORMATION: **Print:** Editors, *Drug & Natural Medicine Advisor: The Complete Guide to Alternative & Conventional Medications,* Time/Life, 1997. **Contact/Web** site: American Botanical Council, PO Box 201660, Austin TX 78720; 1-800-373-7105; www.herbalgram.org. Herb Research Foundation, www.herbs.org.

DHEA (dehydroepiandrosterone)

MANUFACTURERS/BRAND NAME(S): Twinlab, Doctor's A-Z, Enzymatic Therapy, Ultimate Nutrition, Schiff, Kal, Body Ammo, Natrol, among others.

HOW SOLD: As a synthetic or as an animal extract in capsules, sublingual capsules, and tablets, usually 25 mg.

TYPE/DEFINITION: Thermogenic agent. DHEA is a weak androgen, or male hormone, that is present in both sexes. It is produced by the adrenal gland and manufactured from cholesterol, and it is the most abundant hormone in the human bloodstream.

BACKGROUND/RESEARCH: Much research has been done on the anti-aging effects of DHEA, but little has been done in the area of weight loss, except in rats. There are reports that it can help with weight loss, increase sexual energy, reduce memory loss, and treat cancer, diabetes, and Alzheimer's disease, although none of these claims has been proven in humans. Scientists have found, however, that the level of this hormone is highest in adolescence and young adulthood but declines steadily thereafter. This is one of the main reasons it has gained a reputation as an anti-aging compound.

PRODUCT CLAIMS: DHEA has the ability to promote the burning of fat and to increase muscle mass. It does this indirectly by preventing the action of an enzyme that is needed during fat production. The level of DHEA in the body peaks at about age twenty and then steadily declines. This loss of DHEA has prompted many experts to recommend that people take a supplement not only because of its fat-fighting and muscle-building abilities, but because it also appears to help slow the aging process. Some experts claim it also guards against cancer and heart disease and boosts the immune system, but these claims have not been proven.

DOSAGE INFORMATION: The manufacturers' suggested dosage ranges from 5 to 25 mg daily. Some experts recommend having your DHEA levels checked (your doctor can do a blood or saliva test) before you take DHEA supplements.

SIDE EFFECTS: DHEA can cause insomnia; acne; fatigue; irritability; and oily skin; and in women it can also cause facial hair growth and deepening of the voice. Some men report breast enlargement when taking DHEA. Doses higher than 25 mg can cause heart palpitations in some people. The long-term effects of DHEA supplementation are unknown, but may include cancer as discussed below.

PRECAUTIONS: Because DHEA is an androgen, or male sex hormone, anyone with a personal or family history of hormone-related tumors, such as breast, endometrial, or prostate cancer, should not take it. Supplemental DHEA could stimulate the growth of breast and prostate tumors. In fact, studies show high levels of DHEA in women with breast cancer and endometrial cancer. Generally, healthy people younger than forty should not take DHEA because it can hinder the body's ability to produce the hormone naturally. If you are taking estrogen, your dosage may need to be modified if you decide to take DHEA.

FURTHER INFORMATION: Barrett-Connor, E., and Ferrara, A., Dehydroepiandrosterone, dehydroepiandrosterone sulfate, obesity, waist-hip ratio, and noninsulin dependent diabetes in postmenopausal women: the Rancho Bernardo Study. *J Clin Endocrinol Metab*, Jan. 1996, 81(1): 59–64; Usiskin, K. S., et al., Lack of effect of dehydroepiandrosterone in obese men. *Int J Obes*, 1990, 14:457–63; Yen, S. S., et al., Replacement of DHEA in aging men and women: Potential remedial effects. *Ann NY Acad Sci*, 1995, 774:128–42; Yen, T. T., et al., Prevention of obesity in Avy/a mice by dehydroepiandrosterone, *Lipids*, May 1977, 12(65): 409–13. Also see Sahelian, Ray, *All About DHEA*, Avery, 1999; Cherniske, Stephen, *The DHEA Breakthrough*, Ballantine, 1998; Challem, Jack, *The ABCs of Hormones: What You Need to Know About Melatonin, DHEA, Pregnenolone, Sex Hormones, HGH, Insulin, Thyroid, and More*, Keats, 1998.

Ephedra (*Ephedra sinica*)

MANUFACTURERS/BRAND NAME(S): Also known as *ma huang, Mormon tea, cowboy tea, squaw tea, and desert herb*. Although it is not readily available as a single supplement, it is a major ingredient in many popular diet products, such as Metabolife, and herbal fen-phen products, among others.

HOW SOLD: Powder, tincture, tablets, and decoction.

TYPE/DEFINITION: Thermogenic agent, decongestant. Ephedra is an herb that contains a potent substance called ephedrine, which many pharmaceutical companies make in synthetic form and put in over-the-counter drugs to treat respiratory problems, including colds, bronchitis, asthma, and whooping cough.

BACKGROUND/RESEARCH: Ephedra has been the subject of much research and has been found to be potentially dangerous, especially when used for weight loss. A combination of ephedra, green tea, and kola nut, commonly used to raise the metabolic rate and thus help in weight loss, can cause damage to the heart and the nervous system. At least forty people have died and more than 800 have become ill after taking diet products that contain ephedrine, including the sudden death of a college student in 1997. Some states have outlawed the use of ephedra or placed severe restrictions on its use because of its ability to cause serious reactions, as well as increased blood pressure, uncontrolled sweating, and increased blood flow to the brain.

The manufacturers of ephedra products insist that the herb is safe. The FDA, which had been trying to regulate the supplement, is now trying to get warning labels placed on the products.

Strong evidence to support such warning labels appeared in two different reports. In May 2000, scientists noted that many labels of products containing ephedra were not accurate. The researchers checked twenty different brands, and in ten, the amount of active ingredient varied from the stated amount by 20 percent or more. One product did not contain any ephedra, and several brands contained possibly dangerous combinations of ephedra and caffeine and other products.

Another report, published in December 2000, highlighted the potential for serious cardiovascular and central nervous system adverse reactions associated with the dietary supplements that contain ephedra. In the study, 31 percent of the 140 reports of the adverse reactions reported to the Food and Drug Administration between June 1, 1997, and March 31, 1999, were definitely or probably related to use of the supplement, and another 31 percent were possibly related. Of that 62 percent, 47 percent involved cardiovascular symptoms and 18 percent affected the central nervous system. The most commonly reported symptoms were hypertension, palpitations, rapid heartbeat, stroke, and seizures.

However, another study, also made public in December 2000, claimed that ephedra is safe when taken at a dosage of 90 mg to 150 mg 3 times a day. The announcement, made by the Council for Responsible Nutrition, was the result of a study that analyzed nineteen clinical trials of ephedra. The reviewers concluded that ephedra did not cause any adverse reactions at the 90-mg-per-day dose and only minimal side effects at 150 mg per day. According to John Cordano, president and CEO of the Council for Responsible Nutrition, the FDA's reports of problems with ephedra were incorrect because they contained incomplete information, were based on taking the supplement with other products, or the doses taken were too high. He cautioned, however, that anyone who has heart disease; coronary thrombosis; diabetes; glaucoma; hypertension; thyroid disease; poor cerebral circulation; renal problems; an enlarged prostate; or adrenal tumors should not take ephedra.

PRODUCT CLAIMS: Ephedra contains the active ingredients ephedrine, pseudoephedrine, and norpseudoephedrine, which stimulate the cardiovascular and central nervous systems. Ephedrine stimulates the beta receptors in the fat cells, which then turn on the process known as thermogenesis, which burns fat and produces energy.

DOSAGE INFORMATION: Inasmuch as this substance has been associated with or led to the deaths of numerous people and medical problems in many others, it would be irresponsible to offer suggestions for its use, especially when safer alternatives are available. Those alternatives can be found throughout this book.

SIDE EFFECTS: Ephedrine causes heart palpitations; dry mouth; insomnia; headache and dizziness; an increase in blood pressure, metabolic rate, perspiration rate, and urine output; and a reduction of the secretion of stomach acid. In some cases it can cause paranoid psychoses; coronary spasm; convulsions; respiratory depression; coma; and death.

PRECAUTIONS: Never use ephedra or products containing it unless you are under the supervision of a physician. Do not consume coffee, tea, or other caffeinated products when using ephedra. People with heart disease; high blood pressure; thyroid disease; nervous disorders; or poor digestion; who are weak or who experience insomnia or excessive perspiration; who are pregnant or breast-feeding; or who are taking any types of medications, especially those that increase blood pressure, should not use ephedra. If you are over age sixty-five, consult your doctor before using this product.

FURTHER INFORMATION: **Print:** Haller, C. A., and Benowitz, N. L., Adverse cardiovascular and central nervous system events associated with dietary supplements containing ephedra alkaloids. *New Eng J Med* Dec. 21, 2000, 343 (25): 1833–38. Theoharides, T. C., Sudden death of a healthy college student related to ephedrine toxicity from a ma huang–containing drink. *J Clin Psychopharm*, Oct. 1997, 37: 917–22; White, L. M., Pharmacokinetics and cardiovascular effects of ma huang in normotensive adults. *J Clin Pharm,* Feb. 1997.

Fennel (*Foeniculum vulgare*)

MANUFACTURERS/BRAND NAME(S): Nature's Herbs, Nature's Way, Alvita, Frontier, Gaia Herbs, among others.

HOW SOLD: Capsules, tincture, dried seeds, bulk tea.

TYPE/DEFINITION: Appetite suppressant. Its original Greek name was *marathron* from *maraino*, meaning "to grow thin." In Arabian medicine it is used as a diuretic. Fennel is native to the Mediterranean but is now widely cultivated.

BACKGROUND/RESEARCH: The value of fennel as a weight-loss herb is largely anecdotal. It has been used as an appetite suppressant since ancient Greek times. A tradition among people of later centuries was to eat the seeds during Lent to suppress hunger. The seeds, leaves, and roots were made into tea and used by those "that are grown fat, to abate their unwieldiness and cause them to grow more gaunt and lank," according to seventeenth-century British herbalist Nicholas Culpepper. Today fennel is often used to aid digestion and to relieve diarrhea.

PRODUCT CLAIMS: Fennel seeds contain 4 to 6 percent essential oils, 16 to 20 percent protein, and various vitamins, minerals, and sugars. It is believed these compounds help to suppress the appetite, yet exactly how it works is unknown.

DOSAGE INFORMATION: Experts recommend that fennel be taken between meals. To make an infusion, they suggest placing 1 to 3 g crushed or ground seeds in 8 ounces boiling water, steeping them for 15 minutes, and drinking 2 to 3 cups daily. To use the tincture, experts say to add 5 to 15 mL to water and to take this dose 2 to 3 times daily.

SIDE EFFECTS: Fennel is generally regarded as safe. In very rare cases it may cause rash.

PRECAUTIONS: Do not take fennel if you are pregnant or breast-feeding, or if you have a chronic gastrointestinal disease, such as an ulcer, reflux esophagitis, colitis, or diverticulitis. Fennel should be avoided if you have a history of alcoholism; liver disease; estrogen-dependent breast tumors; or abnormal blood clotting. In animal studies, fennel has exacerbated liver damage, but there are no human studies of this effect.

FURTHER INFORMATION: **Print:** European Scientific Cooperative on Phytotherapy (ESCOP), Foeniculi aetheroleum and Foeniculi fructus. *Monographs on the Medicinal Uses of Plant Drugs.* 1997; Tanira, M. O. M., et al., Pharmacological and toxicological investigations on Foeniculum vulgare dried fruit extract in experimental animals. *Phytother Res*, 1996, 10:33–36. **Contact/ Web site:** American Botanical Council, PO Box 201660, Austin TX 78720; 1-800-373-7105; www.herbalgram.org; and Herb Research Foundation, www.herbs.org.

5-HTP (5-hydroxytryptophan)

MANUFACTURERS/BRAND NAME(S): Arizona Natural, Doctor's A-Z, Natrol, among others.

HOW SOLD: Capsules, usually 50 mg.

TYPE/DEFINITION: Amino acid. 5-HTP is a chemical precursor (something that precedes another) of the neurotransmitter serotonin. The supplement 5-HTP is a derivative of the African plant *Griffonia simplicifolia*, which grows in the Ivory Coast and Ghana. The body produces 5-HTP from the amino acid tryptophan, which is found in certain foods, including almonds, turkey, and cheese.

BACKGROUND/RESEARCH: Studies of 5-HTP for weight loss were first done in animals in 1975. At that time, scientists found that feeding 5-HTP to rats that were bred to overeat caused them to eat far less food than they normally ate. These studies led scientists to theorize that some people may be genetically predisposed to obesity because they have a decreased ability to convert tryptophan to 5-HTP, which results in low levels of another substance, called serotonin. Low levels of serotonin are associated with obesity as well as depression.

After the animal studies, three placebo-controlled, double-blind studies in people were conducted in Rome, Italy, which demonstrated the benefits of 5-HTP (see Further Information). One study involved twenty obese women who were told not to diet while they received either 5-HTP or placebo for 6 weeks. Then they were placed on a diet (1,200 calories per day) for 6 weeks while continuing to take 5-HTP or placebo. Women who had taken 5-HTP reduced their caloric intake during the first 6 weeks and reduced their carbohydrate intake by 50 percent. During the second 6-week period, they reduced both their caloric and carbohydrate intake even more. The women who had taken placebos showed very little reduction in caloric intake, even when instructed to diet during the second 6-week period. These findings suggest that 5-HTP reduces cravings for carbohydrates and thus the amount of calories consumed. Another study of nineteen women had similar results: women taking 5-HTP lost weight, even when they did not restrict their caloric intake.

PRODUCT CLAIMS: Researchers believe that 5-HTP may be effective in weight loss because it has the ability to chemically "trick" the brain into thinking you are full soon after you begin to eat, which means you are less likely to overeat and you will consume fewer calories. This theory is associated with the idea that some people have a genetically caused decreased ability to convert tryptophan to 5-HTP, which results in their having decreased levels of the hormone serotonin. Low serotonin levels are associated with obesity; studies have shown that low amounts of this neurotransmitter produce cravings for carbohydrates that can be mild to severe. By taking supplements of 5-HTP, the body's inability to convert tryptophan is bypassed, more serotonin is produced, and the cravings subside.

DOSAGE INFORMATION: Generally, manufacturers suggest taking 50 to 100 mg 5-HTP about 20 minutes before meals during the first 2 weeks. The dosage can be doubled if weight loss is less than 1 pound per week after that time. 5-HTP should always be taken with an adequate amount of vitamin B_6 and zinc (at least the recommended daily intake) because these nutrients help make the 5-HTP more available to the body. A high-quality multivitamin-mineral that supplies at least 25 mg vitamin B_6 and 15 mg zinc is sufficient.

SIDE EFFECTS: Some people experience mild nausea, heartburn, flatulence, and a feeling of fullness in the abdomen. At high doses (more than 300 mg per day) nausea is common. This symptom is usually transitory, but it may take several weeks to disappear.

PRECAUTIONS: Recent research suggests that high blood levels of 5HT (serotonin) may cause damage to the heart muscle and fibrous growths on the aortic valve. This is thought to be what happened to users of fen/phen which also raised serotonin levels. Therefore, people who have cardiovascular disease, such as coronary artery disease, congestive heart failure, pulmonary hypertension, or cardiomyopathy, should not take 5-HTP. If you are taking any type of prescription or over-the-counter medication, talk with your doctor before taking 5-HTP. Potentially serious side effects, such as confusion or anxiety, may occur if you take 5-HTP while taking antidepressants, lithium, buspirone, levodopa, or cold remedies that contain ephedrine or pseudoephedrine. If you are taking antihistamines, muscle relaxants (e.g., carisoprodol, cyclobenzaprine), or narcotic pain relievers, you may experience excessive drowsiness.

FURTHER INFORMATION: **Print:** Birdsall, T. C., 5-hydroxytryptophan: a clinically effective serotonin precursor. *Altern Med Rev*, Aug. 1998 (4): 271–80; Ceci, F., et al., The effects of oral 5-hydroxytryptophan administration on feeding behavior in obese adult female subjects. *J Neural Transm*, 1989, 76: 109–17; Goodwin, G. M., et al., Plasma concentrations of tryptophan and dieting. *BMI*, 1990, 300: 1499–1500; Anderson, I. M., et al., Dieting reduces plasma tryptophan and alters brain 5HT function in women. *Psychol Med*, 1990,

20:785–91; Cangiano, C., et al., Eating behavior and adherence to dietary prescriptions in obese adult subjects treated with 5-hydroxytryptophan. *Am J Clin Nutr*, 1992; 56:863–67. Also see Murray, Michael, N.D., *The Natural Way to Overcome Depression, Obesity and Insomnia*, Bantam, 1999; Sahelian, Ray, M.D., *Nature's Serotonin Solution*, Avery, 1999.

**Garcinia cambogia (hydroxycitric acid);
also known as HCA**

MANUFACTURERS/BRAND NAME(S): Natrol, Nature's Answer, Nature's Plus, Nature's Herbs, Source Naturals, among others. Sold by many manufacturers under different trademarks, including but not limited to CitriMax (trademark of Inter-Health Co.), Citrin, and Citrin K.

TYPE/DEFINITION: Appetite suppressant. Garcinia cambogia is obtained from a pumpkin-shaped Indian fruit of the same name, but eating the fruit, rather than taking the HCA extract, does not cause weight loss. It is also known as malabar tamarind and is occasionally referred to as brindell berry.

HOW SOLD: Tablets, extract, capsules.

BACKGROUND/RESEARCH: In 1991, the first study of the use of HCA for weight loss was done in people; however, the participants were also given chromium picolinate. During the 8-week double-blind study, the people who took HCA and chromium lost an average of 11.1 pounds compared with 4.2 pounds in the placebo group. Two subsequent tests using the same substances came up with similar results—an average of 11 pounds lost in 8 weeks. Whether the weight loss was the result of HCA or chromium alone, or the combination, could not be determined by these studies. At least four other studies using HCA along with one or more other substances, including caffeine and chitosan, show similar loss of weight, but again none of the losses can be attributed to HCA alone.

An obscure case study was published in 1988 in which an individual who ate 1 gram of malabar tamarind before each meal reportedly lost 1 pound per day. The only well-controlled study of HCA used alone for weight loss was done in 1998 and published in the *Journal of the American Medical Association*. In this study, 135 overweight men and women received either HCA or placebo, along with a low-calorie, high-fiber diet. The daily dose of HCA was 1,500 mg (500 mg 3 times a day, 30 minutes before meals). After 3 months, the people taking HCA lost an average of 9 pounds while the placebo group lost an average of 7 pounds. Yet the people in the placebo group lost more body fat than those in the HCA group.

PRODUCT CLAIMS: Exactly how it might help people drop pounds is not known. According to A. A. Conte, who was the investigator in all three studies just mentioned, the combination of HCA and chromium picolinate reduced both appetite and a craving for sweets, as well as reduced fat formation and storage. Some experts say garcinia promotes the storage of excess calories as glycogen, a carbohydrate that the body uses for energy, rather than fat.

DOSAGE INFORMATION: Manufacturers say that HCA should be taken about 30 minutes before meals 3 times a day at a dose of 250 mg.

SIDE EFFECTS: No side effects have been reported.

PRECAUTIONS: No precautions are associated with the use of this substance. It is not known to interact with medications.

FURTHER INFORMATION: **Print:** Conte, A. A., A nonprescription alternative in weight reduction therapy. *The Bariatrician*, summer 1993; Conte, A. A., The Allendale Study, in *Citrin: A Revolutionary, Herbal Approach to Weight Management*. Rosen, R., et al., eds., New Editions, 1994; Conte, A. A., The Hilton Head Study II: Citrin 75, in *Citrin: A Revolutionary, Herbal Approach to Weight Management*. Rosen, R., et al., eds., New Editions, 1994; Conte, A. A., The effects of (−) Hydroxycitrate and chromium (GTF) on obesity. Abstract 50, 35th Annual Meeting of the American College of Nutrition, Atlanta, October 1994; Firenzuoli, F., and Gori, L., Garcinia cambogia for weight loss. *JAMA* July 21, 1999, 282(3): 234; Heymsfield, S. B., et al., Garcinia cambogia (Hydroxycitric acid) as a potential antiobesity agent. *JAMA*, Nov. 11, 1998, 280:1596–1600; Rothacker, D. Q., and Waitman, B. E., Effectiveness of a *Garcinia cambogia* and natural caffeine combination in weight loss: A double-blind placebo-controlled pilot study. *Int J Obesity*, 21 (Supp 2): 53; Sergio, W., A natural food, malabar tamarind, may be effective in the treatment of obesity. *Med Hypothesis,* 1988; 27: 40.

Ginseng (*Panax quinquefolius*); American ginseng (*Eleutherococcus senticosus*); Siberian ginseng

MANUFACTURERS/BRAND NAME(S): Gaia, Nature's Way, Nature's Answer, Zand, among others.

TYPE/DEFINITION: Herb. American ginseng is native to the United States and is now considered to be an endangered species because of overharvesting. Siberian ginseng is found in Russia and has similar but milder effects than American ginseng.

HOW SOLD: Fresh and dried root, capsules, tablets, prepared tea, root powder.

BACKGROUND/RESEARCH: There is evidence that ginseng assists with metabolism when the body is under a lot of stress. Ginseng also acts as a catalyst for energy production. Generally, this herb is not considered to be a weight-reducing supplement on its own, although it does have a minor effect on metabolism and also reduces blood pressure.

PRODUCT CLAIMS: Ginseng is found in many weight-loss combination products and enables the body to better cope with stress, which in turn allows the body to function better. In American ginseng, the compounds believed to be responsible for these activities are panoxosides and saponins, which calm the brain and stomach and act as a mild stimulant to the vital organs. In Siberian ginseng, substances called eleutherosides stimulate the immune system. Generally, Siberian ginseng is less potent than American ginseng, but because American ginseng is considered an endangered species, Siberian ginseng is found more often in products.

DOSAGE INFORMATION: To prepare an infusion, experts say to add 1 tablespoon fresh root to 8 ounces water, simmer for 15 to 20 minutes, and drink up to 2 cups daily. For extracts, they suggest adding 20 to 40 drops to water and drinking this mixture 3 times a day.

SIDE EFFECTS: Ginseng may cause insomnia and agitation, but these symptoms are more common if you take ginseng along with caffeine-containing foods or beverages. Other side effects include headache, breast soreness, rash, and loose stools.

PRECAUTIONS: If any of the following symptoms occur, stop taking ginseng and consult your doctor: elevated blood pressure; asthma attacks; heart palpitations; or postmenopausal uterine bleeding.

FURTHER INFORMATION: **Print:** MoroMarco, Jacques, *The Complete Ginseng Handbook,* NTC/Contemporary Books, 1997; Editors, *Drug & Natural Medicine Advisor: The Complete Guide to Alternative & Conventional Medications,* Time/Life, 1997; Prinzenberg, Ernst, *Ginseng: Stay Young and Vital,* Sterling, 1999; Pedersen, Stephanie, *Ginseng: Energy Enhancer,* DK Pub. Merchandise, 2000. **Contact/Web sites:** American Botanical Council, PO Box 201660, Austin TX 78720; 1-800-373-7105; www.herbalgram.org; Herb Research Foundation, www.herbs.org.

Glucomannan

MANUFACTURERS/BRAND NAME(S): Nature's Way, Natrol, Pristine Konjac, among others.

HOW SOLD: Capsules.

TYPE/DEFINITION: Laxative, appetite suppressant. Glucomannan is extracted from the konnyaku root, which is in the yam family. It is a high-fiber, calorie-free substance that is also a good source of beta-carotene, thiamin, and minerals. Glucomannan is also known as devil's tongue and voodoo lily.

BACKGROUND/RESEARCH: Few studies of glucomannan for weight loss have been done; all of them have included fifty subjects or less and have not been double-blind. In 1984, twenty obese subjects took glucomannan before each meal for 8 weeks and did not change their eating or exercise habits. After 8 weeks the mean weight loss was 5.5 pounds, and cholesterol levels had dropped significantly. Subjects in a 1989 study had even better results: after 8 weeks they lost an average of 8.14 pounds. Severely obese patients in Italy who took part in a 3-month study in 1992 reported that glucomannan was effective and well tolerated. In another Italian study, a group of obese children had positive weight loss and a decline in their cholesterol levels as well.

Glucomannan may also protect against certain cancers as well as help prevent heart attack and stroke in people who have diabetes. Some experts claim glucomannan has these benefits because it prevents the formation of plaque in the blood.

PRODUCT CLAIMS: The Japanese have long believed that glucomannan removes toxins from the body through the digestive tract. For centuries, Asian women have claimed that glucomannan has helped them remain slender. Glucomannan reportedly swells up to 50 times its volume when taken with a large (at least 8 ounces) glass of water, although some manufacturers claim a 200-times increase in volume. The glucomannan then forms an insoluble gum in the stomach, which creates a feeling of fullness. Glucomannan reduces fat content in the blood and relieves constipation.

DOSAGE INFORMATION: A typical dosage is 2 to 3 capsules with 8 ounces of water about 20 minutes before meals. Capsules typically are between 450 and 665 mg.

SIDE EFFECTS: Glucomannan reduces the body's ability to absorb vitamin E and several other nutrients.

PRECAUTIONS: While taking glucomannan, ask your doctor to monitor your nutritional status because glucomannan binds with some nutrients and reduces their absorption. Experts recommend taking a multivitamin-mineral supplement while taking glucomannan.

FURTHER INFORMATION: Biancardi, L., et al., Glucomannan in the treatment of overweight patients with osteoarthrosis. *Curr Ther Res*, 1989; 46: 908–12; Cairella, M., Evaluation of the action of glucomannan on metabolic parameters and on the sensation of satiation in overweight and obese patients. *Clin Ther*, 1995; 146(4): 269–74; Livieri, C., et al., The use of highly purified glucomannan-based fibers in childhood obesity.

Pediatr Med Chir, Mar.–Apr. 1992, 14(2): 195–98; Vitar, P. M., et al., Chronic use of glucomannan in the dietary treatment of severe obesity. *Minerva Med*, Mar. 1992, 83(3): 135–39; Walsh, D. F., et al., Effect of glucomannan on obese patients: a clinical study. *Int J Obes*, 1984, 8(4): 289–93; Wu, J., and Peng, S., Comparison of hypolipidemic effect of refined konjac meal with several common dietary fibers and their mechanisms of action. *Biomed Environ Sci*, 1997, 10(1): 27–37.

Green tea (*Camellia sinensis*)

MANUFACTURERS/BRAND NAME(S): Doctor's A-Z, Nature's Herbs, Good Earth, Alvita, Choice Organic Teas, Traditional Medicinals, Solgar, among others.

TYPE /DEFINITION: Metabolic stimulator and diuretic. Green tea is the least processed form of tea.

HOW SOLD: Prepared tea bags, loose tea, and capsules.

BACKGROUND/RESEARCH: In 1999, scientists in Geneva, Switzerland, compared the ability of green-tea extract, caffeine, and a placebo to increase metabolism and burn fat in overweight individuals. They found that green-tea extract, which contains caffeine as well as other compounds, increases the number of calories and fat burned beyond what caffeine alone can do. Another study, published in the March 2000 issue of *Endocrinology*, found that rats given EGCG (epigallocatechin gallate, a substance found in green tea) had a significant decrease in food intake and body weight. These scientists reported that "green-tea extract . . . could be of value in assisting the management of obesity."

PRODUCT CLAIMS: Green tea, unlike black tea, undergoes minimal processing, which involves slightly steaming and then quickly drying the tea leaves. This method allows the green tea to keep its beneficial substances called polyphenols. One type of polyphenol is catechin, and the special catechin in green tea that promotes the burning of fat is called EGCG. Green tea also contains caffeine, which is both a stimulant and a diuretic. These substances work together to promote weight loss.

DOSAGE INFORMATION: Experts believe an effective amount of catechins for weight management is 300 mg. The average cup of green tea contains 50 to 100 mg catechins; thus, depending on the potency of the tea you buy, experts recommend 3 to 6 cups of tea per day. If the green tea you buy only gives the polyphenol level, the amount of catechins is usually lower. You can roughly determine the catechin content by using the following example: To achieve 300 mg of catechin from an extract, you need approximately 480 mg of a 50:1 green-tea extract that contains 60 percent catechin (60 percent of 480 =300 mg).

SIDE EFFECTS: Because it contains caffeine, green tea may cause insomnia, restlessness, irritability, and heart palpitations if taken in excessive amounts.

PRECAUTIONS: Limit your use of green tea if you have a sensitive stomach, heart problems, an overactive thyroid, or kidney problems. Do not use green tea if you are pregnant or breast-feeding. Too much green tea (more than 1.5 g per day) over a long time can cause insomnia, dizziness, heart palpitations, and irritability. Also avoid green tea if you are taking alkaline drugs, such as antacids and most antidepressants and prescription painkillers.

FURTHER INFORMATION: **Print:** Dulloo, A. G., et al., Green tea and thermogenesis: interactions between catechin-polyphenols, caffeine and sympathetic activity. *Intl J Obesity*, Feb. 2000, 24 (2): 252–58; Dulloo, A. G., et al., Efficacy of a green tea extract rich in catechin polyphenols and caffeine in increasing 24-h energy expenditure and fat oxidation in humans. *Am J Clin Nutr*, Dec. 1999, 70 (6): 1040–45; Kao, Y. H. et al., Modulation of endocrine systems and food intake by green tea epigallocatechin gallate. *Endocrinology*, Mar. 2000, 141 (3): 980–87; Taylor, Nadine, *Green Tea: The Natural Secret for a Healthier Life*, Kensington, 1998.

Guar gum (*Cyamopsis tetragonoloa*)

MANUFACTURERS/BRAND NAME(S): Natrol, Source Naturals, among others.

TYPE/DEFINITION: Guar gum is a complex carbohydrate that is

derived from the seed pods of the guar tree, which is native to India and grown in the southwest United States. It is used as a laxative.

HOW SOLD: Capsules and dietary fiber.

BACKGROUND/RESEARCH: Guar gum is an approved emulsifier and a common additive to foods, such as low-fat cheeses and other low-fat dairy products. It was used in diet products until 1992, when the FDA banned its use in nonprescription diet products because several people experienced a blockage of their esophagus and gastrointestinal tract after using the product incorrectly. Investigators later found that the people who had these blockages had not drunk enough liquids when taking the guar gum. With the passage of the 1994 Dietary Supplement Health and Education Act, however, guar gum is now generally recognized as safe (GRAS).

The clinical studies that have looked at guar gum have been small but have shown positive results. Three were done in the 1980s and involved a total of thirty-seven subjects. At a dose of 20 grams per day, nine subjects lost an average of 9.4 pounds over 2 months, 21 lost 15.6 pounds over 2½ months, and 7 lost 61.9 pounds over 1 year. A fourth study reported in 1994 showed an average loss of 5.5 pounds over 2 months while taking 15 grams per day.

PRODUCT CLAIMS: When guar gum makes contact with liquids, it forms a heavy, viscous mass, which makes people feel full. It also hinders fat absorption from the intestines.

DOSAGE INFORMATION: Manufacturers always recommend taking guar-gum supplements with a full 8 ounces of water. A typical dosage for capsules is up to four 500 mg daily. The usual dosage for the powder is 1 teaspoon in 8 ounces of liquid 1 to 3 times daily.

SIDE EFFECTS: No side effects when taken as directed. See Precautions.

PRECAUTIONS: If you take guar-gum supplements with an insufficient amount of liquid, the gum may swell in your throat and cause a blockage. Always take the supplement with at least 8 ounces of water.

FURTHER INFORMATION: **Print:** Anonymous, Better than oat bran. *Science News*, 1994; 145:28; Ide, T., et al., Hypolipidemic effects of guar gum and its enzyme hydrosylate in rats fed highly saturated fat diets. *Annals of Nutr and Metab*, 1991, 35: 34–44; Krotkiewski, M., Effect of guar gum on body weight, hunger ratings and metabolism in obese subjects. *Br J Nutr*, 1984; 52: 97–105; Krotkiewski, M., Effect of guar on body weight, hunger ratings and metabolism in obese subjects. *Clin Sci*, 1984, 66: 329–36; Okubo, T., et al., Effects of partially hydrolyzed guar gum intake on human intestinal Microflora and its metabolism, *Biosci Biotech Biochem*, 1994, 58 (8): 1364–69; Takahashi, H., et al., Effect of partially hydrolyzed guar gum on fecal output in human volunteers, *Nutr Res* 1993, 13:649–57.

Guarana (*Paullinia cupana*)

MANUFACTURERS/BRAND NAMES(S): Natrol, Nature's Answers, among others.

TYPE/DEFINITION: Thermogenic agent. Guarana is a creeping shrub that grows in the Amazon. It bears small, bright red fruit that contains a black seed, which is the part of the plant used for medicinal purposes.

HOW SOLD: Powder, syrup, capsules, tincture.

BACKGROUND/RESEARCH: Most of the evidence that guarana helps with weight loss is anecdotal. Many South American Indian tribes, especially the Guaranis, for whom this plant is named, use guarana as a stimulant. It is the primary ingredient in a popular Brazilian beverage called Guarana Soda.

Studies in animals and in humans have suggested that guarana increases physical endurance and memory, and that it has antibacterial qualities.

PRODUCT CLAIMS: Guarana seeds contain several substances that appear to be responsible for its weight-loss properties. One is tetramethylxanthine (present at a level of up to 5.8 percent), a substance that is nearly identical to caffeine. When ingested, this caffeinelike compound is released slowly in the body over 4 to 6 hours, so the energy boost it gives is unlike the dramatic quick peak caffeine causes. Substances called saponins seem to be one reason guarana has this long-lasting effect.

Two other stimulating ingredients found in guarana, but in much smaller amounts, are theobromine and theophylline. Theobromine is the stimulant found in chocolate, and theophylline is a related compound. It is only mildly stimulating and is used to treat asthma. Together these three compounds stimulate the body's metabolism.

DOSAGE INFORMATION: To use the tincture, manufacturers suggest adding ½ to 1 mL tincture to water 2 to 3 times a day. For capsules (usually 200 mg), the typical dosage is 1 to 2 once a day with water, either before breakfast or before lunch. Directions for preparing powders and syrups vary by manufacturer. Avoid taking guarana late in the day, as it may cause insomnia.

SIDE EFFECTS: When used as recommended, no serious side effects have been reported. Because it has caffeinelike qualities, guarana may cause insomnia, trembling, anxiety, urinary frequency, and heart palpitations. Long-term use may cause a decline in fertility and cardiovascular disease.

PRECAUTIONS: In 1998, the FDA conducted a test of fourteen over-the-counter products that claimed to contain guarana. The agency reported that "a number of these products may not contain authentic guarana as an active ingredient or contain less than the declared quantity of guarana." If you plan to purchase guarana, look for a reliable, well-established manufacturer.

Guarana is not recommended if you are pregnant, as it may harm the fetus, or if you have heart disease.

FURTHER INFORMATION: **Print:** Carlson, M., et al., Liquid chromatographic determination of methylxanthines and catechins in herbal preparations containing guarana. *J AOAC Int*, Jul.–Aug. 1998, 81(4): 691–701; Galduroz, J. C., and Carlini, E. A., The effects of long-term administration of guarana on the cognition of normal, elderly volunteers. *Rev Paul Med*, Jan.–Feb. 1996, 114:1073–78; Mindell, Earl, *Earl Mindell's Herb Bible*, Simon & Schuster, 1992; van Straten, Michael, *Guarana: The Energy Seeds & Herbs of the Amazon Rainforest*, CW Daniel, 1995. Miura, T., et al., Effect of guarana on exercise in normal and epinephrine-induced glycogenolytic mice. *Biol Pharm Bull*, Jun. 1998, 21(6): 646–48. **Web sites:** http://guarana.homepage.com and www.symmetrix.ch/Public/guarana/index.html.

Guggul (*Commiphora mukul*)

MANUFACTURERS/BRAND NAME(S): Nature Care, Frontier, Enzymatic Therapy, Natrol, among others.

HOW SOLD: Capsules, tablets.

TYPE/DEFINITION: Thermogenic agent. Guggul is the purified and standardized resin derived from the mukul tree, which grows in India.

BACKGROUND/RESEARCH: Guggul is an Indian Ayurvedic herb that has been used for weight management for more than 2,000 years. Most of the evidence concerning its effectiveness for weight loss is anecdotal and steeped in Ayurvedic tradition. During the 1960s, however, a researcher named G. V. Satyavati studied the herb extensively for two years and submitted her findings to what was then the College of Medical Sciences, Banaras Hindu University. Together with Professor C. Dwarakanath, she conducted experiments in rabbits and found that guggul significantly lowered the amount of fats, including cholesterol, in the bloodstream and reduced body weight. Subsequent studies in obese adults also reduced cholesterol levels.

Chemists later identified two components in guggul that seemed to provide the most benefit, E-guggulsterone and Z-guggulsterone. However, guggul also contains many other compounds, including lignans, sterols, and fatty acid alcohols, and many researchers believe they all work synergistically to produce its various benefits.

PRODUCT CLAIMS: The guggulsterones in guggul increase the secretion of thyroid hormone in rats and improve the ability of the gland to absorb iodine. Iodine is essential for the production of the thyroid hormone. Stimulation of the thyroid helps the body burn calories more efficiently and thus contributes to weight loss.

DOSAGE INFORMATION: Herbalists recommend looking for extracts that contain 5 to 10 percent guggulsterones. The suggested dosage of guggulsterones is 25 mg 3 times daily. Do not use guggul for more than 6 months.

SIDE EFFECTS: Guggul is believed to be very safe when used as directed. However, if it does work by stimulating the thyroid gland and thus the metabolic rate, this can have harmful effects, particularly in individuals with heart disease. Guggul also may cause mild abdominal discomfort in some people who use it long term.

PRECAUTIONS: Because safety of guggul in people with severe liver or kidney disease has not been established, consult your physician before using guggul if you have either of these conditions.

FURTHER INFORMATION: **Print:** Mester, L., et al., Inhibition of platelet aggregation by guggul steroids. *Planta Med*, 1979, 37:367–69; Nityanand, S., and Kapoor, N. K., Hypocholesterolemic effect of *Commiphora mukul* resin (guggul). *Indian J Exp Biol*, 1971, 9:367–77; Satyavati, G. V., Gum guggul (*Commiphora mukul*)—The success of an ancient insight leading to a modern discovery. *Indian J Med*, 1988, 87:327–35.

Gymnema (*Gymnema sylvestre*)

MANUFACTURERS/BRAND NAME(S): Nature Care, among others.

HOW SOLD: Capsules, standardized to at least 25 percent gymnemic acids.

TYPE/DEFINITION: Appetite suppressant. Gymnema sylvestre is a member of the milkweed family and is native to tropical areas of India.

BACKGROUND RESEARCH: Although gymnema sylvestre is often promoted as a weight-loss supplement and is found in many combination weight-loss products, there is only anecdotal evidence to support that claim. A few studies have been done, however, showing how gymnema helps reduce blood-sugar levels, which is helpful for people with diabetes, most of whom are overweight. In one study, twenty-seven people with insulin-dependent diabetes were able to reduce their need for insulin after taking gymnema-leaf extract for several months. Studies in animals have shown that gymnema can double the number of insulin-producing cells in the pancreas and thus help restore blood-sugar levels to normal.

PRODUCT CLAIMS: Gymnema sylvestre has been nicknamed the "sugar destroyer" because when the leaves are chewed, they block the activity of the sweet-detecting taste buds on the tongue. This effect only occurs when the leaves are chewed, however; taking a capsule or other form of the herb does not change the taste in a person's mouth or reduce the craving for sugar.

In Ayurvedic medicine, gymnema sylvestre is believed to help remove excess sugar from the body, which is said to be the result of an imbalance in the body's doshas. (In Ayurvedic philosophy, there are three basic types of human constitution, or doshas: vata, pitta, and kapha. Remedies are often recommended based on a person's dosha.) Gymnema sylvestre reduces blood cholesterol and blood fat levels.

DOSAGE INFORMATION: Manufacturers generally suggest taking 200 mg 2 times daily.

SIDE EFFECTS: No side effects have been reported when gymnema is taken as directed.

PRECAUTIONS: No precautions have been noted.

FURTHER INFORMATION: **Print:** Baskaian, K., et al., Antibiotic effect of a leaf extract from Gymnema sylvestre in noninsulin-dependent diabetes mellitus patients. *J Ethnopharmacol*, Oct. 1990, 38 (3): 295–300; Shanmugasundaran, E. R., et al., Use of Gymnema sylvestre leaf extract in the control of blood glucose in insulin-dependent diabetes mellitus. *J Ethnopharmacol*, Oct. 1990, 30(3): 281–94; Wang, L. F., et al. Inhibitory effect of gymnemic acid on intestinal absorption of oleic acid in rats. *Can J Physiol Pharmacol*, Oct.–Nov. 1998, 76(10–11): 1017–23.

Human growth hormone (hGH) enhancers (over-the-counter)

MANUFACTURERS/BRAND NAME(S): HGH Enhancer, by Nature's Rx; Ultra HGH, Biotropin (spray), PRO-hGH Symbiotropin by Nutraceutics, among others.

TYPE/DEFINITION: Human growth hormone (hGH) enhancers are over-the-counter products that provide various substances that are known to stimulate the body's own production of human growth hormone, a naturally occurring hormone manufactured and secreted by the pituitary gland. In humans and other mammals, natural human growth hormone is the main hormone responsible for protein synthesis, fat metabolism, and growth. Do not confuse hGH enhancers with the prescription from of hGH, which is a synthetic, injectable product originally developed to treat undersized children with a deficiency of growth hormone. It doesn't make adults grow. However, because hGH is viewed as an anti-aging supplement by some people, some adults are getting injections of the very expensive prescription hGH from their doctors to fight the aging process and to help with weight loss. The discussion here focuses primarily on OTC hGH enhancers.

HOW SOLD: Spray, powder, wafers.

BACKGROUND/RESEARCH: The development of hGH enhancers was prompted partly by research that showed the impact that supplementation with synthetic hGH has on body fat. For example, in 1990, Daniel Rudman, M.D., published his study findings on the impact of supplementation with human growth hormone in older men. In the *New England Journal of Medicine* article, he noted that "diminished secretion of growth hormone is responsible in part for the decrease in lean body mass, the expansion of adipose-tissue (fat) mass, and the thinning of the skin that occurs in old age." At the end of the 6-month study, Rudman saw a 14.4 percent loss of body fat even though the participants had not made any change to their diet or exercise programs. Overall, some research shows that supplementation with growth hormone causes a 5 to 10 percent increase in lean body mass and a 5 to 18 percent decrease in fat tissue.

Another study, published in 1991, showed success when treating obese women with human growth hormone. In the double-blind, placebo-controlled study, twelve women were divided into two groups: six received hGH and six received placebo 3 times a week for 4 weeks. At the end of the study, the hGH group had a significant reduction in body fat without having reduced their caloric intake; the placebo group had no reduction.

PRODUCT CLAIMS: The hGH enhancers work by supplying the body with compounds known to increase the body's natural manufacturing of hGH. It is known that people who are overweight have low levels of growth hormone secretion, but researchers do not know the reason for this decrease. They do know, however, that the body's normal production of growth hormone is modulated by various factors, including stress, nutrition, exercise, aging, sleep, and two hormones: growth hormone releasing hormone (GHRH) and somatostatin. The various hGH enhancers on the market contain different substances that affect the actions of GHRH and somatostatin (e.g., the amino acids glutamine and arginine), as well as the actions of other substances that have an impact on these two hormones.

DOSAGE INFORMATION: Typically package directions suggest the sprays be administered under the tongue, 2 to 3 sprays several times a day, and that the powder be taken on an empty stomach because hGH levels rise when insulin levels are low. An hGH enhancer also should be taken with a minimal amount of water (3 to 4 ounces) because water dilutes it.

SIDE EFFECTS: The only side effect reported is mild joint pain lasting 1 to 2 months when you first begin taking the supplement. However, excess growth hormone causes insulin resistance and can thus cause diabetes or aggravate preexisting diabetes. Therefore, it must be used with caution in people with diabetes or persons at risk for diabetes, which includes overweight individuals.

PRECAUTIONS: Do not take hGH enhancers if you have cancer; thyroid dysfunction; enlarged prostate; high blood pressure; hypothyroidism; hypocortisolemia; or hypoglycemia; or if you are pregnant, trying to get pregnant, or are breast-feeding.

FURTHER INFORMATION: **Print:** Azain, M. J., et al., Effect of somatotropin and feed restriction on body composition and adipose metabolism in obese Zucker rats. *Am J Physiol,* July 1995,

269(1, pt. 1): E137–E144; Kanaley, J. A., et al., Human growth hormone response to repeat bouts of aerobic exercise. *J Appl Physiol*, Nov. 1997, 83(5): 1756–61; Klatz, Ronald, *Grow Young with hGH*, HarperPerennial, 1998; Rudman, Daniel, Effects of human growth hormone on men over 60 years old. *New Eng J Med*, July 5, 1990, 323(1): 1–6; Skaggs, S. R., and Crist, D. M., Exogenous human growth hormone reduces body fat in obese women. *Horm Res*, 1991, 35(1): 19–24; *HGH: Human Growth Hormone*, Woodland Publishing, 1999; Winter, Ruth, *The Anti-Aging Hormone that Can Help You Beat the Clock: Benefits and Dangers of Melatonin, Human Growth Hormone, DHEA, Estrogen, Testosterone, Insulin, and Others*, Crown, 1997. **Web site**: www.reverseaging.net.

Kola nut

MANUFACTURERS/BRAND NAME(S): Zand, Herb Pharm, Nature's Answer.

TYPE/DEFINITION: Thermogenic agent and diuretic. The kola nut is the seed kernel of the African kola tree. It is also known as bissy nut.

HOW SOLD: Capsules, extract.

BACKGROUND/RESEARCH: Evidence that kola nut helps with weight loss is largely anecdotal. One animal study found that body weight decreased in rats that had received 18 weeks of kola-nut supplement. Studies in humans, however, are lacking.

PRODUCT CLAIMS: Kola nut contains caffeine, theobromine, and tannins, which stimulate the metabolism and urinary excretion.

DOSAGE INFORMATION: To use the extract, experts suggest adding 10 to 15 drops to water and taking it 2 to 3 times a day. Package directions typically suggest taking 1 to 2 capsules daily.

SIDE EFFECTS: Because kola nut contains caffeine, insomnia, tremors, heart palpitations, and nervousness may occur.

PRECAUTIONS: Do not take kola nut if you are pregnant or breast-feeding. Before taking kola nut, consult your doctor if you are taking any medications or have high blood pressure, heart or thyroid disease, or a nervous disorder.

FURTHER INFORMATION: **Print:** Ikegwuonu, F. I., et al., Effects of kola-nut extract administration on the liver, kidney, brain, testis and some serum constituents of the rat. *J Appl Toxicol*, Dec. 1981, 1(6): 292–94.

Kelp (*Fucus vesiculosus*) (also known as seaweed or bladderwrack)

MANUFACTURERS/BRAND NAME(S): Nature's Herb, Frontier, Nature's Way, among others.

TYPE/DEFINITION: Sea vegetable. Often the terms kelp, seaweed, and bladderwrack are used interchangeably, which is not entirely accurate as there are many types of seaweed, of which kelp and bladderwrack are but two. However, they all are a source of iodine, which is the main reason seaweed is taken for weight loss. Some products listed in Part III have more than one type of seaweed listed in their ingredients; however, the differences among them are minor.

HOW SOLD: Capsules (typically around 640 mg), dried, extract, powder, lotion.

BACKGROUND/RESEARCH: Most of the evidence that kelp is helpful in weight loss is anecdotal. The results of an Italian study published in 1976 showed that people who took kelp lost more weight than those who did not take the seaweed. The majority of research on kelp, however, has concerned the possibility that it inhibits the development of breast cancer, and how it can be used in the treatment of digestive problems and bronchial congestion.

PRODUCT CLAIMS: Because an underactive thyroid can lead to weight gain and lethargy, some people take kelp to promote weight loss and to enhance their energy level. Kelp contains iodine, which helps regulate thyroid function. Kelp contains polysaccharides, which stimulate the immune system. Some researchers claim that kelp increases the metabolic rate by raising hormone production created by the thyroid. Kelp also acts as a mild diuretic. There have also been reports that a topical form of kelp can eliminate cellulite. However, as yet there is no firm evidence that kelp helps in weight loss or in eliminating cellulite.

DOSAGE INFORMATION: Package directions usually suggest taking kelp between meals. To prepare an infusion, experts recommend steeping 1 heaping teaspoon of dried kelp in 8 ounces hot water for 30 minutes and drinking 1 cup 1 hour before each meal and 1 cup before retiring. Capsules should be taken with food. To use the extract, package directions typically advise adding 30 to 40 drops to water and taking it 3 times a day.

SIDE EFFECTS: Kelp is usually safe if taken according to package directions.

PRECAUTIONS: Large doses of kelp may induce hyperthyroidism or it may make existing cases of the disease worse. Consult your doctor if you are taking iodine-containing medications. Look for kelp that has been harvested from deep ocean waters or from near the Arctic Circle—that is, as far removed from polluted waters as possible.

FURTHER INFORMATION: **Print:** *Monograph: Bladderwrack*, Milan, Indena SpA, 1987.

Maitake (*Grifola frondosa*)

MANUFACTURERS/BRAND NAME(S): Nature's Answer, Grifon Maitake, Planetary Formulas, Nature's Herbs, among others.

TYPE/DEFINITION: Mushroom. It is grown in Japan, where it is called the "dancing mushroom" because people reportedly danced for joy when they found this mushroom in the wild.

HOW SOLD: Tablets, capsules, tincture.

BACKGROUND/RESEARCH: In Japanese studies that have involved humans and rats, maitake mushroom has promoted weight loss. In one study, thirty human participants lost an average of 11 to 13 pounds after taking maitake daily for 2 months without changing their diet. Studies with rats had similar results.

PRODUCT CLAIMS: Studies suggest that the fruit body of maitake helps regulate body weight and cholesterol levels.

DOSAGE INFORMATION: Typical manufacturers' dosages are 1 to 2

500-mg capsules or tablets 3 times daily, or 1 mL (about 28 drops) of 1:2 tincture 2 times daily. Take maitake between meals.
SIDE EFFECTS: There are no side effects associated with this mushroom.
PRECAUTIONS: No known precautions are necessary. Maitake does not appear to interact with medications.
FURTHER INFORMATION: **Print:** Ohtsura, H., Anti-obesity activity exhibited by orally administered powder of maitake mushroom (*Grifola frondosa*). *Anshin*, July 1992, 198. Yokoto, M., Observatory trial at anti-obesity activity of maitake mushroom (*Grifola frondosa*). *Anshin*, July 1992, 202. Kubo, K., and Nanba, H., The effect of maitake mushrooms on liver and serum lipids. *Altern Ther Health Med*, Sept. 1996, 2(5):62–66.

Medium-Chain Triglycerides (MCTs)

MANUFACTURERS/BRAND NAME(S): Ultimate Nutrition.
TYPE/DEFINITION: Medium-chain triglycerides are a type of fatty acid. They differ from other fats in that they are water soluble and are absorbed more rapidly, even in people with conditions that impair their digestion of other fats. Medium-chain triglycerides are sometimes referred to as caprylic acid or capric acid.
HOW SOLD: Tablets, capsules.
BACKGROUND/RESEARCH: Investigators have found that medium-chain triglycerides increase calorie burning when compared with other types of fat. However, they also discovered that people would need to eat 50 percent of their calories as medium-chain triglycerides for significant weight loss to occur. They discovered this after doing a study in which 24 percent of the total calories were consumed as medium-chain triglycerides, and the participants did not experience any greater weight loss than subjects who ate other types of fat.
PRODUCT CLAIMS: Medium-chain triglycerides seem to work best when they are added to a carbohydrate solution and when they are taken at very high amounts—namely, 50 percent of total calories. However, most experts agree this amount is

unrealistic for the majority of people, and likely will not result in any significant weight loss.

DOSAGE INFORMATION: Until further research studies have been conducted, experts do not know the best amount of MCTs to take. Current manufacturers recommend taking 1 tablespoon with meals or using it instead of cooking fats and oils in recipes. Medium-chain triglycerides are for individuals who want to change their body composition. It may or may not result in weight loss.

SIDE EFFECTS: Taking MCTs on an empty stomach causes gastrointestinal upset.

PRECAUTIONS: Medium-chain triglycerides should not be used if you have diabetes, acidosis, or any type of liver disorder. A by-product of MCT metabolism is the formation of ketone bodies, which are harmful to diabetics. MCTs are delivered rapidly to the liver and can be too stressful for people with liver disease. Several reports suggest that MCTs may raise triglyceride and cholesterol levels, but more study is needed.

FURTHER INFORMATION PRINT: Bach, A. C., et al., The usefulness of dietary medium-chain triglycerides in body weight control: fact or fancy? *J Lipid Res*, 1996; 37:708–26; Scalfi, L., et al., Postprandial thermogenesis: in lean and obese subjects after meals supplemented with medium-chain and long-chain triglycerides, *Am J Clin Nutr*, 1991, 53:1130–33; Yost, T. J., and Eckel, R. H., Hypocaloric feeding in obese women: metabolic effects of medium-chain triglyceride substitution. *Am J Clin Nutr*, 1989, 49:326–30.

Omega-6 (gamma-linolenic acid or GLA)

MANUFACTURERS/BRAND NAME(S): Natrol, Rainbow Light, Source Naturals, Spectrum Naturals, Health From the Sun, among others.

TYPE/DEFINITION: An essential fatty acid that acts as a metabolic stimulator. It has a critical role in the production of hormone-like substances called prostaglandins, which perform various important functions in the body.

HOW SOLD: GLA is found in evening primrose oil, borage oil, and black currant oil, all of which are available in capsules or softgels. Evening primrose oil is the most common of the three oils. When purchasing evening primrose oil, look for a product that contains 35 to 40 mg GLA per 500-mg capsule.

BACKGROUND/RESEARCH: Several studies suggest that GLA promotes weight loss in individuals who have not lost weight while following appropriate reduced-calorie plans. But in a 12-week, double-blind study of seventy-four obese women, researchers found that those women who took evening primrose oil did not lose significantly more weight than the women who were given a placebo.

PRODUCT CLAIMS: There is a type of fat called brown fat, which plays a role in the conversion of food into energy. There is speculation that when people consume excessive amounts of food, a rapid conversion of brown fat takes place as a way to balance out an overproduction of white fat, which makes up the majority of fat on the body. Some experts believe that this conversion process is compromised in some people and leads to obesity. Thus, they propose that supplementing with GLA may help stimulate brown-fat activity, thereby increasing fat metabolism.

According to Dr. Elson M. Haas, author of *Staying Healthy with Nutrition*, theoretically GLA raises cell metabolism and helps maintain the water and electrolyte balance in the body.

DOSAGE INFORMATION: According to experts, the recommended daily doses of GLA can be achieved by taking either of the following 2 to 3 times per day: 500 to 1,000 mg of borage oil or evening primrose oil, or 100 to 200 mg of black currant oil.

SIDE EFFECTS: No side effects have been reported when GLA is used as directed.

PRECAUTIONS: No precautions have been assigned to GLA.

FURTHER INFORMATION. **Print:** Haslett, C., et al., A double-blind evaluation of evening primrose oil as an antiobesity agent. *Int J Obes*, 1983, 7(6): 549–53. Also see Haas, Elson M., M.D., *Staying Healthy with Nutrition*, Celestial Arts, 1992.

Parsley

MANUFACTURERS/BRAND NAME(S): Nature's Herb, Select Teas, Gaia Herbs, among others.

TYPE/DEFINITION: Diuretic. Parsley is a member of the carrot family.

HOW SOLD: Dried root, prepared tea bags, capsules, tincture, fresh.

BACKGROUND/RESEARCH: Most of the evidence supporting the use of parsley for weight loss is anecdotal. Traditionally, it has been used for centuries to treat water retention, menstrual cramps, and insect bites.

PRODUCT CLAIMS: Scientists have identified many of the substances in parsley but are not exactly certain how they give this herb its helpful qualities. They know that parsley's chlorophyll content is responsible for its ability to freshen the breath, and they believe its essential oil, which contains apiol, myristicin, and terpenes, may be responsible for some of its other properties, including increased urination. The leaves are a rich source of vitamin C and flavonoids, and the roots are a good source of protein, vitamins, minerals, and flavonoids.

DOSAGE INFORMATION: To make an infusion, herbalists suggest adding 1 teaspoon to 8 ounces boiling water, allowing it to steep for 15 minutes and drinking it 3 times a day. A typical dosage for capsules is two 400- to 450-mg capsules 2 to 3 times daily with meals. Experts note that the contents of the capsules can also be used to make tea. When using the tincture, a typical dosage is 30 to 40 drops in warm water taken up to 3 times a day.

SIDE EFFECTS: Side effects are rare; they may include dizziness, photosensitivity, nausea, and vomiting.

PRECAUTIONS: Do not use parsley if you are pregnant or breastfeeding, as it can cause uterine contractions. People with kidney problems should avoid parsley because it can stress the organ.

FURTHER INFORMATION. Print: Feyes, S., et al., Investigation of the in vitro antioxidant effects of Petroselinum crispum (Mill.) Nymex AW Hill. *Acta Pharm Hung*, 1998, 68 (3): 150–56.

Phenylalanine (L-phenylalanine)

MANUFACTURERS/BRAND NAME(S): Source Naturals, Twinlab, among others.

TYPE/DEFINITION: L-phenylalanine is a nonessential amino acid, which means the body produces it. It is similar in its chemical structure to phenylpropanolamine (PPA), which has been removed from the market for safety reasons, but differs in how it affects the brain.

HOW SOLD: Tablets, capsules, typically 500 mg. Phenylalanine comes in three forms: L- , D- , and DL-phenylalanine. The L-form is the most common and is the one that may be helpful for obesity.

BACKGROUND/RESEARCH: The treatment of depression is one of the main uses for L-phenylalanine. However, studies show that L-phenylalanine levels are low in people who are obese, which suggests that supplementation with this amino acid may help with weight loss.

PRODUCT CLAIMS: Phenylalanine may suppress appetite because it promotes the production of cholecystokinin (CCK), a neurotransmitter that signals the body to stop desiring food.

DOSAGE INFORMATION: Experts disagree on how to use L-phenylalanine and whether it is an effective appetite suppressant. Some researchers recommend taking 100 to 500 mg before retiring; others say to take it before each meal. In either case, experts recommend *never* taking L-phenylalanine for longer than 3 weeks without a break and only taking it while under medical supervision.

SIDE EFFECTS: At high doses (1,500 mg or more), L-phenylalanine can cause anxiety, increased blood pressure, and headache. Report any side effects immediately to your doctor.

PRECAUTIONS: Do not take L-phenylalanine if you are pregnant or nursing, if you get migraines, if you are allergic to food proteins (e.g., wheat, eggs, and meat), or if you have diabetes, high blood pressure, or phenylketonuria (PKU, an inability to process L-phenylalanine). Avoid L-phenylalanine if you have existing malignant melanoma cells, as this amino acid can promote cell division. Taking L-phenylalanine supplements may cause an amino-acid imbalance or eye lesions. Therefore, it is best to take a general amino-acid supplement along with L-phenylalanine to help maintain amino-acid balance in the body.

FURTHER INFORMATION. **Print:** Greenwood-Robinson, M., Natural fat burners team up, *Let's Live*, Jan. 2000, 1:28.

PPA: OFF THE MARKET

In September 2000, the FDA sent a memorandum to Charles Ganley, M.D., director of the Division of Over-The-Counter Drug Products, and recommended that products containing PPA (phenylpropanolamine hydrochloride) "no longer be available over the counter." Some of these dietary products included Acutrim, Dexatrim, Dexatrim Extra Duration, Propagest, and Westrim, which have now been discontinued or reconstituted. (PPA was also found in many over-the-counter cold and cough remedies. They were included in the warning as well.) This recommendation came soon after a research group studied 702 patients and 1,376 control volunteers from forty-three different centers. The men and women, eighteen to forty-nine years old, reported on their use of cold and cough products and dietary supplements that contained PPA. The scientists found that there is an increased risk of hemorrhagic stroke for women after taking dietary products containing PPA, and possibly cold and cough remedies as well. Men, none of whom reported taking dietary supplements containing PPA, did not demonstrate the same increased risk. The study, headed by W. N. Kernan, M.D., and entitled Phenylpropanolamine and the risk of hemorrhagic stroke, was published in the *New England Journal of Medicine*, 2000: 343, 1826–32.

Psyllium

MANUFACTURERS/BRAND NAME(S): Nature's Way, Nature's Herbs, Metamucil, others.

TYPE/DEFINITION: Husks from the seeds of the psyllium plant are ground into a source of soluble fiber with a variety of effects and uses discussed below.

HOW SOLD: Seeds, powdered husks (loose), in capsules, and as the laxative Metamucil®.

BACKGROUND/RESEARCH: Few studies have examined the role psyllium plays in weight loss, but many have explored its benefits in people with high cholesterol and other fats. These latter studies have shown that fiber, and in particular psyllium, helps reduce cholesterol and fat levels in the blood. In particular, a meta-analysis of sixty-seven studies done by researchers at Harvard School of Public Health found that psyllium, as well as oat bran, guar gum, and pectin, reduced cholesterol and fat levels. Psyllium also slows the digestion and absorption of carbohydrates, which can improve blood-sugar levels in diabetics.

PRODUCT CLAIMS: Psyllium is rich in fiber and a jellylike substance called mucilage. When psyllium makes contact with water, the mucilage absorbs the fluid, which in turn creates a feeling of fullness. This may help reduce appetite.

DOSAGE INFORMATION: Herbalists' suggested daily dose is 1 teaspoon of the husks or up to 2 teaspoons of the powdered seed, which are stirred into an 8-ounce glass of water and drunk immediately before it thickens. Drink plenty of fluids (preferably water) throughout the day.

SIDE EFFECTS: Psyllium is usually safe when taken as recommended, but it can cause abdominal cramps, bloating, and flatulence in some people.

PRECAUTIONS: Take psyllium at different times than other supplements, and do not take with water-soluble supplements (e.g., the B vitamins or vitamin C). Psyllium should always be taken with lots of water, both when taking the supplement and throughout the day. People who have a bowel obstruction should not take psyllium.

FURTHER INFORMATION. **Print:** Brown, L., et al., Cholesterol-lowering effects of dietary fiber: a meta-analysis. *Am J Clin Nutr*, Jan. 1999, 69(1): 30–42; Jenkins, D. J., et al., Viscous fibers, health claims, and strategies to reduce cardiovascular disease risk. *Am J Clin Nutr*, Feb. 2000, 71 (2): 401–2; Neal, G. W., and Balm, T. K., Synergistic effects of psyllium in the dietary treatment of hypercholesterolemia. *South Med J*, Oct. 1990, 83(10): 1131–37; Slap, J. K., Effects of psyllium on serum lipids. *Am J Clin Nutr*, 1998, Oct., 68(4): 923–24.

Pyruvate

MANUFACTURERS/BRAND NAME(S): Natrol, Bodyonics, Kaizen, Twinlab, among others.
TYPE/DEFINITION: Thermogenic agent. Pyruvate is an acid that plays an important role in the metabolism of carbohydrates, proteins, and fats.
HOW SOLD: Capsules, tablets, available in 500-, 750-, and 1,000-mg potencies.
BACKGROUND/RESEARCH: Some studies show that pyruvate lowers cholesterol in individuals who eat a high-fat diet. It also improves cardiac function and improves exercise performance mostly by enhancing the transport of glucose into muscle cells. One researcher reports that pyruvate increased energy levels by 18 percent and reduced fatigue by 71 percent, two situations that help in weight loss.

In a 6-week, double-blind, placebo-controlled study of twenty-six overweight adults, those who took 6 g per day of pyruvate and exercised 3 days per week lost significantly more body fat than subjects who took placebo and also exercised. Over the 6-week period, the participants lost an average of 4.8 pounds of body fat, but their body weight did not change because they gained lean body mass. The researchers stress that "the real enemy is body fat and not just weight." This is a concept that bodybuilders and athletes more readily accept than those who want to lose weight and not just body fat.

There are claims that pyruvate prevents fat regain and the

yo-yo effect whereby dieters lose and regain weight again and again. This claim is based on a single study that was done in a highly controlled environment in which participants lost weight when placed on a 310-calorie-a-day starvation diet. This drastic reduction in calories was followed by a high-calorie diet supplemented with 15 g pyruvate and 75 g dihydroxyacetone (a substance produced by the body that it then converts into pyruvate). The subjects who received the supplement gained less weight (36 percent less, or 3.96 pounds) and less fat (55 percent, or 1.76 pounds) than the untreated group. The dramatic circumstances of the study and the fact that dihydroxyacetone was added make it difficult to determine if pyruvate alone had a role in the amount of weight regained. It also should be noted that the majority of research on pyruvate and weight loss has been done by one research team.

PRODUCT CLAIMS: Pyruvate is the product of a process in which pyruvic acid, an unstable substance, is stabilized by conversion into a salt called pyruvate. This conversion takes place when manufacturers of pyruvate combine the acid with calcium, sodium, potassium, or magnesium. Pyruvate stimulates metabolism and the utilization of fat. Although the reason is not entirely clear, pyruvate also seems to prevent the "plateau" that often occurs after people have been dieting for several weeks. To avoid that plateau, it is necessary to increase the normal daily dosage by about four times.

DOSAGE INFORMATION: Research suggests that pyruvate should be taken before meals or before exercise sessions. According to a University of Kansas study, two 15-minute exercise sessions per day better help people lose weight than one 30-minute session. This is because there is an increase in excess post-exercise oxygen consumption, which translates into more calories burned after each short session than after one long session. Although this study did not specifically mention the use of pyruvate, some experts claim that taking this supplement before each exercise session can increase the amount of calories burned.

SIDE EFFECTS: No side effects have been noted when pyruvate is taken as directed.

PRECAUTIONS: Megadoses (more than ten times the recommended dose) have been shown to cause diarrhea and flatulence.
FURTHER INFORMATION: **Print:** Ivy, J. L., et al., Effects of pyruvate on the metabolism and insulin resistance of obese Zucker rats. *Am J Clin Nutr*, 1994, 59:331–37; Kalman, D., et al., The effects of pyruvate supplementation on body composition in overweight individuals. *Nutrition*, May 1999, 15(5): 337–40; Stanko, R. T., et al., Pyruvate supplementation of a low-cholesterol, low-fat diet: effects on plasma lipid concentrations and body composition in hyperlipidemic patients. *Am J Clin Nutr*, Feb. 1994, 59(2): 423–37; Stanko, R. T., et al., Body composition, energy utilization, and nitrogen metabolism with a 4.25-MJ/d low-energy diet supplemented with pyruvate. *Am J Clin Nutr*, 1992, 56:630–35; Stanko, R. T., et al., Body composition, energy utilization, and nitrogen metabolism with a severely restricted diet supplemented with dihydroxyacetone and pyruvate. *Am J Clin Nutr*, 1992, 55:771–76; Stanko, R. T., and Arch, J. E., Inhibition of regain in both weight and fat with addition of 3-carbon compounds to the diet with hyperenergetic refeeding after weight reduction. *Int J Obes Relat Metab Disord*, Oct. 1996, 20(10): 925–30. Also see Prokop, David, *The Pyruvate Phenomenon: The Facts, the Benefits, the Unanswered Questions*, Woodland, 1999; Stanko, Ronald, *The Power of Pyruvate: The Natural Way to Better Health and Well-Being*, Keats, 1999.

Senna (*Cassia angustifolia*)

MANUFACTURERS/BRAND NAME(S): Alvita, Frontier, Nature's Way, Seelect Teas, among others.
TYPE/DEFINITION: Laxative. Senna is derived from the leaves of a shrub cultivated in northern Africa, India, and the Middle East.
HOW SOLD: Capsules, tablets, extract, tea.
BACKGROUND/RESEARCH: The use of senna as a laxative goes back before 1000 A.D. Reportedly an ancient Egyptian papyrus in the sixteenth century B.C. mentions senna as being prescribed by physicians for the elite.
PRODUCT CLAIMS: Senna contains compounds called senno-

sides, which stimulate the intestinal tract. When it comes to weight loss, at best senna can cause a temporary loss of water weight.

DOSAGE INFORMATION: Senna is recommended for severe constipation, and not as a weight-loss aid. For the extract, experts recommend taking ½ to 1 teaspoon once daily for no more than 3 days. Experts warn that if you use the tea, do not drink more than 2 cups per day for up to 3 days.

SIDE EFFECTS: If senna is used along with a diuretic, such as caffeine, guarana, uva ursi, or tea, it can cause violent diarrhea, severe cramps, dehydration, nausea, vomiting, and electrolyte imbalance (loss of the minerals calcium, magnesium, and potassium). This can be especially dangerous for people who have heart problems.

PRECAUTIONS: Do not use senna for more than 3 consecutive days. Long-term use of senna can lead to dependence on laxatives. Chronic use can also cause reversible clubbing of the fingers and toes, loss of appetite, and serious nutritional deficiencies, as well as discoloration of the lining of the colon and laxative-induced diarrhea. At least one study has found a "cancer-promoting effect of chronic sennoside use." Do not use senna if you are pregnant or nursing. Senna passes into breast milk and may cause diarrhea in breast-fed infants.

FURTHER INFORMATION: **Print:** van Gorkom, B. A., et al., Influence of a highly purified senna extract on colonic epithelium. *Digestion*, 2000, 61(2): 113–20.

Spirulina (*Spirulina maxima* and *Spirulina platensis*)

MANUFACTURERS/BRAND NAME(S): Earthrise, Nature's Way, Nutrex, among others.

TYPE/DEFINITION: Spirulina is a blue-green algae rich in protein, B vitamins, calcium, potassium, magnesium, manganese, iron, selenium, and zinc. It contains all eight essential amino acids. It is considered to be a whole food, not an herb.

HOW SOLD: Tablets, capsules, flakes.

BACKGROUND/RESEARCH: Evidence that spirulina is beneficial for weight loss in humans is largely anecdotal. No scientific studies have been done on spirulina and weight loss in humans. However, animal studies indicate that spirulina may help enhance the immune system, reduce cholesterol levels, and increase energy.

PRODUCT CLAIMS: Unsubstantiated reports say that spirulina suppresses the appetite by increasing the level of **phenylalanine** (an amino acid; see entry, pp. 96–97) in the body. Some experts claim that the combination of chlorophyll, the essential amino acids, vitamins, minerals, and gamma linolenic acid found in spirulina is responsible for its ability to decrease body weight.

DOSAGE INFORMATION: A typical dose of the flakes is 1 to 2 tablespoons per day, dissolved in water or juice. Because spirulina has a strong taste, many people find it easier to drink in a thick juice, like tomato or pear nectar, or in a low-fat soymilk shake. It can also be stirred into yogurt.

SIDE EFFECTS: Occasionally spirulina may cause allergic reactions, such as nausea or vomiting. Discontinue use and consult your doctor.

PRECAUTIONS: If spirulina is grown in polluted or contaminated water, it may contain trace or higher levels of harmful organisms or toxic substances, such as mercury and toxic metals. It is best to buy spirulina only from reputable sources.

FURTHER INFORMATION: **Print:** Becher, E. W., et al., Clinical and biochemical evaluations of the alga spirulina with regard to its application in the treatment of obesity. A double-blind cross-over study. *Nutr Rep Intl*, 1986, 33:565–73; Charmorro, G., et al., Pharmacology and toxicology of spirulina alga. *Rev Invest Clin*, 1996, 48(5): 389–99; Henrikson, R., *Earth Food Spirulina. How this remarkable blue-green algae can transform your health and our planet*, Ronore Enterprises, 1997; Johnson, P. E., and Shubert, L. E., Accumulation of mercury and other elements by spirulina (cyanophyceae). *Nutr Rep Intl*, 1986, 34(6): 1063–71; Miranda, M. S., et al., Antioxidant activity of the microalga Spirulina maxima. *Med Biol Res*, Aug. 1998, 31(8): 1075–79. Also see Challem, Jack, *Spirulina: The Microscopic Nutrient Powerhouse and How It Protects and Restores Health*, Keats, 1982.

Uva ursi (*Arctostaphylos uva-ursi*)

MANUFACTURERS/BRAND NAME(S): Gaia Herbs, Nature's Herbs, Nature's Way, Nature's Answer, Herb Pharm, among others.

TYPE/DEFINITION: Diuretic. Uva ursi is derived from the leaves of the bearberry plant, which grows throughout the northern hemisphere.

HOW SOLD: Tincture, solid extract, capsules, dried leaves.

BACKGROUND/RESEARCH: The evidence that uva ursi is helpful for weight loss is anecdotal. However, it has been used to successfully treat urinary-tract problems for at least 1,000 years around the world.

PRODUCT CLAIMS: Uva ursi contains two phytochemicals, ursolic acid and isoquercetin, that stimulate urinary output. However, the increase is reportedly so mild that it has little effect on loss of water weight. However, it is often included in combination weight-loss products.

DOSAGE INFORMATION: Uva ursi is primarily used to treat urinary-tract infections. When taken for that purpose, the suggested dosage is 1 to 2 teaspoons dried leaves per 8 ounces hot water, steeped for 5 to 10 minutes. Three cups per day is the maximum recommended dose. Do not eat acidic foods (e.g., fruit juice with vitamin C) when taking uva ursi because it upsets the alkaline environment in which the herb works.

SIDE EFFECTS: Uva ursi may turn your urine green, which is harmless. Some people experience stomach upset because of the herb's tannin content.

PRECAUTIONS: Prolonged use can cause liver damage. Do not use this herb if you are pregnant because it may stimulate uterine contractions, or if you are breast-feeding. If you experience ringing in the ears, nausea, or convulsions, stop taking the herb immediately.

FURTHER INFORMATION: **Print:** Matsuda, H., et al., Pharmacological studies on leaf of *Arctostaphylos uva ursi* (L) Spreng. *J Pharm Soc*, 1992; 112:673.

PART III

Combination Weight-Loss Products

IF YOU'VE been looking for a weight-loss or diet product recently, you've probably noticed the vast number of items from which to choose. Although having a big selection can be good, it can also be very confusing. The information in the following part can dispel that confusion.

So many manufacturers have flooded the market with combination weight-loss products; it is impossible to list them all here. However, this part contains a representative sample of those products, including meal-replacement items (which work by replacing a regular, high-calorie meal with a restricted-calorie product such as a shake or food bar) and dieter's teas. Many of the products on the market are similar. For example, there are dozens of weight-loss tablets or capsules that contain chromium picolinate, chitosan, garcinia cambogia, or ephedra. Some have a little more of one ingredient than another; sometimes the milligrams per dose are the same among several brands.

Because there is a great deal of similarity among the many brand-name weight-loss products, this part presents a cross section of what's available in stores, mail order, and on the Internet. If you have a particular product in mind but you do not find it here, chances are excellent that you will find one that is very similar.

BUYER BEWARE

Manufacturers are in business to make a profit, so they need to convince you to buy their merchandise. Thus, they advertise supported by research, and may or may not be true. They include explanations you may see on the package, in advertisements, on Web sites, or other avenues that promote the product.

- **Comments** includes recommendations and suggestions based on research of the product or its ingredients. This entry also includes information about side effects and precautions to consider if you take the product. The presentation of this information is solely for the purpose of helping you make a more informed decision and in no way is meant to be an endorsement of the product.
- **Further Information** generally refers you to the manufacturer's Web site address and, in a few cases, other materials about the product, if available.

A FEW WORDS ABOUT DIETER'S TEAS

There are various teas on the market designated for dieters. These products typically contain one or more of the following natural laxatives: cascara, buckthorn, aloe, senna, rhubarb root, and castor oil. Two of these herbs—*senna and buckthorn—are especially potent and should be used with caution.*

The Food and Drug Administration has received numerous reports of adverse effects associated with the use of various dieter's teas, *including four deaths* that have been attributed to their use. Therefore, the FDA urges consumers to follow package directions carefully when using dieter's teas. Such teas should not be steeped longer than recommended, as stronger teas can cause side effects.

Sometimes the presence of these natural laxatives is not evident from the ingredient list because alternate names are given. Senna, for example, is also known as locust root (see **Senna**, pp. 101–102). If you see the name of an herb or ingredient you do not recognize, look it up. This book can help you identify such substances.

Herbal laxatives are often used as weight-loss aids because

many consumers believe they prevent calories from being absorbed and they are eliminated in the stool. Studies by the FDA's Food Advisory Committee, however, show that diarrhea induced by laxatives has very little effect on weight loss or the absorption of calories. That's because laxatives do their work in the colon and not in the small intestine, where calories are absorbed.

Adverse effects associated with incorrect use of dieter's teas are as follows:

- Short-term: People who use dieter's teas for the first time are the ones most likely to experience these effects, which include stomach cramps, nausea, vomiting, and diarrhea that last several days.
- Chronic: People who use dieter's teas for months or years can experience chronic diarrhea, pain, and constipation caused by a dependency on laxatives.
- Severe: Adverse effects such as fainting, irregular heartbeat, dehydration, electrolyte imbalance, and even death may occur in individuals who use these teas along with a drastic weight-loss program, such as very-low-calorie diets, or are anorectic or bulimic. The four deaths reported to the FDA were in this category, and all the women involved had a history of such medical problems.

A FEW WORDS ABOUT HERBAL EXTRACTS

Several of the entries contain the term "standardized" extracts and places where herbal extracts are given in ratios. Here is what these terms mean.

Standardized extracts are the concentrated dried residue of the fluid derived (extracted) from an herb. Standardized extracts are preferred over regular extracts because they are more potent and they provide a "standard" herbal product that maintains its quality from batch to batch, which means you are guaranteed the same potency time after time. Therefore, you may see "St. John's wort (standardized 0.3 percent hypericin)," which means the product is guaranteed to contain the active ingredient hypericin at 0.3 percent, which happens to be the acceptable percentage for St. John's wort.

An extract may be presented as a ratio—say, 40:1—which means the concentrated extract is 40 times stronger than the whole herb. Therefore, if a capsule contains 150 mg of ginseng, for example, and the ratio given is 40:1, that is equivalent to taking 6,000 mg of the whole herb. You get the benefit of 6,000 mg of whole herb in only 150 mg of standardized extract.

GUIDELINES FOR BUYING COMBINATION WEIGHT-LOSS PRODUCTS

As a quick review, keep the following guidelines in mind when buying combination weight-loss products.

- More is not always better. An impressive list of ingredients in a proprietary blend can mean little or nothing because you have no way of knowing exactly what you are getting and how much.
- Make sure any reportedly effective ingredients are present at adequate levels to promote weight loss. For example, in Part II you learned that the reported beneficial dose of chromium picolinate is 200 to 400 mcg per day for women. If the product you are considering contains 10 mcg chromium picolinate along with a proprietary blend of eight or ten substances in undisclosed amounts, that product may not be helpful to you.
- Consider safety. Does the product contain ingredients that are unsafe? Are you taking any medications or using other substances (e.g., alcohol, caffeine) that are dangerous to use with this product? Are you allergic to any of the ingredients, including fillers? If you have any doubt at all about combining a diet product with any-

thing you are currently taking, consult with your physician before starting the weight-loss product.

- Are the dosage instructions ones you can easily follow? If you need to take the product every few hours or if taking it conflicts with your schedule or other medications you take, you should look for a more convenient product.

- Beware of products that "require" you to buy several or an entire line of dietary merchandise. This tactic can lock you into an expensive, inconvenient, and unrealistic weight-loss program.

- Always read labels, even if you have bought the product previously. Manufacturers often make ingredient changes or modifications to their instructions, warnings, or other information. Such a change may not be obvious, especially if the label or packaging itself has not changed in any noticeable way.

- Read between the lines of all the advertising materials that accompany each product. Look for ambiguous and weak statements; you won't have to look far in many cases. "Studies prove" and "research shows" are good only if the manufacturer can back up their claims with unbiased studies, which means they were not done or funded by the manufacturer.

BEST BETS

Minolest: The three ingredients (glucomannan, guar gum, and psyllium) in this product have been shown to produce satiety and help reduce appetite in some people. It is safe when used as directed.

Satietrol: The two primary ingredients, glucomannan and guar gum, have been shown to produce satiety and help reduce appetite in some people. No adverse effects have been reported when used as directed.

SlimFast: This product is a reasonable meal replacement if it

---

BEST BETS (*Cont.*)

is used as directed; that is, *it should not be the sole source of nutrition*, and the other one or two regular meals should be healthy ones.

Weight Loss Plus Green Tea: Scientific studies have shown that green tea boosts metabolism. Green tea is the primary ingredient in this product, and the other ingredients are considered to be safe.

Aoqili Slim Soap

ACTION: Fat-reducing soap.

HOW SOLD: Bars; imported from China and available through U.S. distributors.

INGREDIENTS: Aoqili Slim Soap is made from "the elixirs of under-sea plants, including rare seaweeds." Other unnamed ingredients include trace elements, vitamins, and minerals. The manufacturer claims the soap is based on ancient Chinese medicine.

DOSAGE INFORMATION: The manufacturer says Aoqili should be used in the shower, *not a bath*. The package instructions are to rinse your entire body and hair, allowing the pores to open. With your back to the shower, lather the front of your body. For each part of the body you wish to slenderize, grasp that area and massage it with the lather for a count of 60. Repeat on the next area you wish to slenderize. Users are encouraged to drink lots of water every day.

PRODUCT CLAIMS: Aoqili reportedly begins to work after 5 days as its "defatting agents" penetrate the skin and enter the fat cells and help reduce them. The package labeling claims that the soap can "discharge the underskin fat out of human bodies." In addition to helping you lose inches, it reportedly also enhances skin texture, enriches the hair, and hardens the nails.

According to an independent empirical study by Professor Masami Asayama at Chukyo University in Aichi Prefecture, Japan, eight women lost an average of 0.2 kg (1/10 of a pound) over a 3-month period. They also lost 2.3 mm (just under 1 inch) from their upper arms, 0.8 mm (0.32 inch) from their back, and 4.2 mm (1.68 inches) from their abdomen. Despite these extremely small results, advertisements for Aoqili also claim tremendous weight loss. The Chinese Council of Science and Technology sponsored a study of the soap and reported that the 433 subjects lost 22 to 110 pounds, and 76 percent lost an average of 33 pounds. There is no indication, however, of what other weight-loss methods these people were using at the same time.

COMMENTS: There is no scientific basis for any of the claims made by the manufacturer or the researchers. The only claims that appear to be true are that Aoqili reportedly is very mild and does not irritate even very sensitive skin.

FURTHER INFORMATION: **Print:** Marshall, Samantha, It's so simple: just lather up, watch the fat go down the drain, *Wall Street Journal*, November 2, 1995. **Web sites:** The product is available at various sites, including www.dfwbiznet.com and www. infohwy.com.

Apple Cider Vinegar with Centella, by Ageless Company

ACTION: Stimulates metabolism, suppresses the appetite.

HOW SOLD: Liquid.

INGREDIENTS: Apple cider vinegar is made from fresh apples and contains chlorine, calcium, iron, magnesium, potassium, sulfur, sodium, silicon, and centella. Centella (*Centella asiatica*) is also known as pennywort or wild violet and is native to Africa, India, and Australia. The ancient Indians ate the leaves to ward off aging.

DOSAGE INFORMATION: The manufacturer recommends mixing 2 level dessert spoons (about 4 teaspoons) of bran with 2 teaspoons of Apple Cider Vinegar with Centella and adding this mixture to oatmeal, yogurt, or fruit and eating it in the morning.

PRODUCT CLAIMS: The advertisements claim that Apple Cider Vinegar with Centella is used around the world to suppress appetite, detoxify the body, boost the immune system, and aid metabolism in burning food effectively. Because this product contains the fiber pectin, the manufacturer says it also helps eliminate cholesterol and reduces high blood pressure. This product is also reportedly helpful with varicose veins and skin lesions because it has an effect on the collagen matrix and the support structure in the skin.

COMMENTS: There are no reliable scientific studies to support the claims made about this product.

FURTHER INFORMATION: **Print:** Bragg, Paul C., et al., *Apple Cider Vinegar: Miracle Health System*, Health Science, 1998. **Web site:** www.ageless.co.za.

AS-200 and PM-300, by AMS

ACTION: A-200 stimulates the metabolism; PM-300 strengthens the immune system.

HOW SOLD: Caplets.

INGREDIENTS: The AS-200 product contains citrin (**garcinia cambogia [HCA]**), 500 mg; **chromium picolinate**, 200 mcg; biotin, 150 mcg; brindell berry, 500 mg; folic acid, 400 mcg; **green-tea** extract, 50 mg; niacinamide, 20 mg; pantothenic acid, 10 mg; vitamin A, 10,000 IU; vitamin B_1 (thiamine hydrochloride), 1.5 mg; vitamin B_2 (riboflavin), 1.7 mg; vitamin B_6 (pyridoxine hydrochloride), 2.0 mg; vitamin B_{12} (cyanocobalamin), 6.0 mcg; vitamin C, 500 mg; and white willow bark, 100 mg. The PM-300 is advertised as a "melatonin complex" that contains, in addition to melatonin, valerian root, lemon balm leaf, scullcap, peppermint leaf, hops, chamomile flowers, kava kava, pantothenic acid, biotin, vitamin C, vitamin A, green-tea extract, brindell berry, and white willow bark. The formula is proprietary.

DOSAGE INFORMATION: The manufacturer recommends taking AS-200 along with PM-300. The suggestion is to take 1 to 3 PM-300 caplets after breakfast and 1 to 3 AS-200 caplets at various times during the day to curb cravings.

PRODUCT CLAIMS: Reportedly, chromium reduces cravings for sugar and carbohydrates and helps reduce fat cells; citrin and the B vitamins suppress the appetite. Citrin (HCA) also reportedly causes glucose to convert to glycogen instead of breaking down into fat or cholesterol. It does this by inhibiting citrate lyase, an enzyme in the liver that regulates fat metabolism. Green tea supposedly regulates blood-sugar levels, and white willow bark has a calming effect.

COMMENTS: The main ingredients in AS-200—**chromium** and **HCA**—have not been proven to promote weight loss. The PM-300 contains a variety of herbs that are commonly used for their calming effect, including valerian root, hops, and chamomile. However, whether this combination of products will result in weight loss is highly questionable.

Although AS-200 can be taken with other medications, it is best to consult your doctor before you take this or any herbal product. Do not take AS-200 or PM-300 if you are pregnant or breast-feeding. If you have diabetes and are taking insulin or any antidiabetic medications, consult your physician before taking this or any product that contains chromium. Chromium has the ability to lower insulin resistance, alter the type or amount of medication needed to control diabetes, and change the frequency with which blood-sugar monitoring should be done.

FURTHER INFORMATION: **Web site:** www.weight-free-lifestyles. com/as_200.htm.

Biodrine, by Biogenics 2000™

ACTION: Stimulates metabolism, suppresses appetite.
HOW SOLD: Capsules.
INGREDIENTS: Four capsules contain **ephedra**, 276 mg; **L-carnitine**, 100 mg; white willow bark, 100 mg; quercetin, 100 mg; HCA (**garcinia cambogia**), 1,000 mg; potassium, 100 mg; magnesium, 100 mg; **guarana**, 1,000 mg.
DOSAGE INFORMATION: Package directions advise taking 2 capsules 2 times a day with meals.
PRODUCT CLAIMS: Of the primary ingredients, HCA helps suppress appetite and hinder the production of cholesterol and fat; L-carnitine oxidizes and transports fatty acids and helps increase good cholesterol levels; and guarana and ephedra stim-

ulate metabolism. This product is advertised as being for people who want to lose weight without consuming a large amount of ephedrine; however, typical **ephedra** doses are about 90 mg per day, so this product actually contains three times the usual dose. COMMENTS: This product contains **ephedra**, which has been linked with serious side effects, including death. It also contains a caffeine-containing substance, **guarana**. This combination is likely to cause anxiety, insomnia, agitation, and other reactions. See entries in Part II for details, pp. 67–70 and 82–84.
FURTHER INFORMATION: **Web site:** See http://discountnutrition.com and www.pro-hormone.com.

Caloloss, by Nature's Plus

ACTION: Assists natural weight loss.
HOW SOLD: Two-phase program that includes tablets and liquid.
INGREDIENTS: The Caloloss AM formula is a two-layered tablet. The rapid-release layer contains **garcinia cambogia** extract (standardized 60 percent HCA), 250 mg; **chitosan**, 100 mg; **L-carnitine**, 50 mg; LipoZyme (a proprietary complex of lipase, protease, amylase, and apple cider vinegar), 50 mg; **chromium** (polynicolate and picolinate), 100 mcg. The sustained-release layer contains a proprietary blend of willow bark (9 percent salicin); **green tea** (50 percent polyphenols); gingerroot (4 percent volatile oils); ashwaganda (1.5 percent withanolida); Siberian **ginseng** (0.8 percent eleutherosides); **cayenne** (minimum 60,000 heat units); along with Super Citrimax (**garcinia cambogia,** 60 percent HCA), 100 mg; and Lipotrop-Ultra (proprietary complex of PeptideFM [patented, bioactive oligopeptides] and niacinamide), 15 mg.

The Caloloss PM formula contains the amino acids in the following Optimal Collagen Profile: alanine, 10.8; valine, 2.3; leucine, 2.7; isoleucine, 1.2; proline, 13.2; phenylalanine, 1.5; methionine, 0.4; glycine, 32.7; aspartic acid, 4.8; glutamic acid, 7.6; lysine, 2.9; hydroxylysine, 0.5; arginine, 5.4; serine, 2.9; hydroxyproline, 8.2; threonine, 1.9; tyrosine, 0.4; and histidine, 0.6. The other ingredients in the liquid are purified water; fructose; collagen hydrolysate; vegetable glycerin; natural cherry flavor; potassium sorbate; and citric acid.

DOSAGE INFORMATION: Package instructions advise taking 2 of the tablets with 8 ounces of water with the morning meal and ¾ tablespoon (12 ml) of the PM formula immediately before retiring with 8 ounces of water on an empty stomach.

PRODUCT CLAIMS: The manufacturer claims this two-phase weight-management program assists with the body's natural weight-loss process. It combines the benefits of soluble collagen amino acids with a blend of botanical extracts which, along with a low-fat diet and exercise, can result in weight loss.

COMMENTS: This program provides a complete amino-acid supplement, which you may or may not need, depending on your diet and other supplements you may be taking. Its usefulness as a weight-loss aid is highly questionable.

If you are pregnant or breast-feeding, consult your doctor before starting this program. If you have diabetes and are taking insulin or any antidiabetic medication, consult your physician before taking this or any product that contains chromium. Chromium has the ability to lower insulin resistance, alter the type or amount of medication needed to control diabetes, and change the frequency with which blood-sugar monitoring should be done.

FURTHER INFORMATION: **Web site:** Available on several Internet sites, including www.mothernature.com.

ChitoGenics, by New Life

ACTION: Absorbs fat and suppresses appetite.
HOW SOLD: Tablets.
INGREDIENTS: **Chitosan,** 300 mg from shellfish; **ephedra,** 150 mg; **kola nut,** 100 mg; ascorbic acid (vitamin C), 50 mg; and pantothenic acid, 10 mg. Proprietary ingredients include **garcinia cambogia** (HCA), **gymnema,** white willow powder, and gingerroot powder.
DOSAGE INFORMATION: A typical dosage is 1 to 2 tablets 30 minutes before meals.

PRODUCT CLAIMS: Chitosan reportedly absorbs fat, and garcinia cambogia (HCA) blocks the conversion of carbohydrates to fat and suppresses the appetite. Both ma huang (ephedra) and kola nut stimulate metabolism. It is uncertain whether the proprietary ingredients are present at levels sufficient to be effective.

COMMENTS: This product contains **ephedra**, which has been linked with serious side effects, including death. It also contains **chitosan,** whose proposed benefits are under scrutiny (see **Chitosan** in Part II, pp. 52–55). Do not take ChitoGenics if you have heart problems, thyroid disease, diabetes, or are allergic to shellfish.

FURTHER INFORMATION: **Web site:** See www.oneononenutrition. com.

Chromium Reducing Formula, by Earth Science

ACTION: Reduces appetite.

HOW SOLD: Liquid extract.

INGREDIENTS: One ml contains chromium picolinate, 200 mcg; vitamin B_6, 5 mg; bladderwrack (**kelp**), 50 mg; vitamin E, 10 IU; **garcinia cambogia,** 50 mg; zinc, 2 mg. Chromium Reducing Formula does not contain any starch, yeast, corn, soy, dairy, sugar, wheat, or artificial colors, flavors, or preservatives.

DOSAGE INFORMATION: According to the manufacturer, add 1 dropper (1 ml) to a small amount of water, juice, or other liquid 3 times a day, 30 minutes before meals.

PRODUCT CLAIMS: Chromium picolinate is claimed to reduce cravings, garcinia cambogia reduces appetite, and bladderwrack stimulates metabolism. The extract is in a base of purified water and natural flavors.

COMMENTS: There is no reliable scientific evidence to support the manufacturer's claims. If you want to take garcinia to help you lose weight, note that the amount of garcinia in the recommended daily dose of this product is significantly lower than the 750 mg reported to effectively suppress appetite.

If you have diabetes and are taking insulin or any antidiabetic medications, consult your physician before taking this or any product that contains chromium. Chromium has the ability to lower insulin resistance, alter the type or amount of medication needed to control diabetes, and change the frequency with which blood-sugar monitoring should be done.

FURTHER INFORMATION: **Web site:** See www.gaines.com.

Citrus Diet, by NaturaLab

ACTION: Stimulates metabolism, burns fat.

HOW SOLD: Capsules.

INGREDIENTS: Two capsules (one serving) contain: vitamin B_6, 40 mg; **chromium** chelate, 200 mcg; potassium carbonate, 50 mg; **citrus aurantium**, 320 mg; ma huang **(ephedra)** (8 percent extract), 250 mg; **garcinia cambogia** (50 percent HCA), 300 mg; **guarana** (22 percent extract), 100 mg; white willow bark, 100 mg; **kelp** (*focus vesiculosus*), 80 mg; **cascara sagrada**, 80 mg; **uva ursi** (*arctostaphylos*), 50 mg; lecithin, 50 mg; **cayenne**, 30 mg; licorice root (*glycyrrhiza glabra*), 30 mg; vanadium (celate), 100 mcg; gingerroot, 30 mg.

DOSAGE INFORMATION: Per package directions, take 2 capsules with water before meals.

PRODUCT CLAIMS: Of the main ingredients, chromium reportedly helps reduce sugar and carbohydrate cravings; citrus aurantium, ma huang, guarana, white willow bark, and cayenne stimulate metabolism; garcinia cambogia suppresses appetite; cascara sagrada is a laxative; and uva ursi is a diuretic.

The literature says Citrus Diet was "created to help millions of people to manage their weight without the difficulties of a diet." The ingredients "have been selected from literally thousands of possible components to create the most favorable combination." Citrus Diet is advertised as an energy booster, a fat burner, and a tool for weight management.

COMMENTS: This product contains several potentially harmful ingredients, including ma huang **(ephedra)**, which is associated with serious side effects, including death; and **cascara sagrada**. See individual entries in Part II for details. If you have diabetes and are taking insulin or any antidiabetic medications, consult your physician before taking this or any product that contains chromium. Chromium has the ability to lower insulin resistance, alter the type or amount of medication needed to control diabetes, and change the frequency with which blood-sugar monitoring should be done.

FURTHER INFORMATION: Citrus Diet is part of a multilevel marketing program. **Web site:** www.naturalab.com.

C-U-Loss, by Herbalife

ACTION: Promotes urination.

HOW SOLD: Tablets.

INGREDIENTS: Three tablets contain vitamin C, 250 mg; potassium, 297 mg; iron, 9 mg; lecithin, 50 mg; **kelp**, 100 mg; cider vinegar, 100 mg; and a proprietary blend totaling 1,000 mg containing buchu, corn silk, hydrangea, juniper berry, couch grass, and **uva ursi**.

DOSAGE INFORMATION: A typical dosage is 1 tablet 3 times a day with meals. The manufacturer notes that for maximum results, C-U-Loss should be taken along with other Herbalife weight-loss products.

PRODUCT CLAIMS: Herbalife claims that C-U-Loss helps decrease the appearance of cellulite and "seems to help drain excess fluid out of fat pockets and cleanses toxins out of cells. Helps promote inch loss immediately."

COMMENTS: The manufacturer does not supply any evidence for its claims. However, based on the ingredients, the herbs in the proprietary blend are diuretics, which may result in minimal, temporary weight reduction due to water loss, and lecithin helps disperse fats in the body's fluids. Also see details about **uva ursi** in Part II, p. 104.

FURTHER INFORMATION: **Web site:** See www.herbalife.com.

Cuts II Xtra Strength, by Prolab Nutrition

ACTION: Weight management.

HOW SOLD: Tablets.

INGREDIENTS: **L-carnitine,** 1,100 mg; lecithin, 1,000 mg; choline, 1,000 mg; inositol, 1,000 mg; methionine, 400 mg; vitamin B$_6$, 80 mg; linoleic acid, 200 mg; oleic acid, 100 mg; **parsley,** 400 mg; potassium gluconate, 400 mg; **chromium picolinate,** 200 mcg; chlorophyll, 4,000 mcg; and grapefruit powder, 200 mg. Also includes a proprietary blend (1,200 mg) of **uva ursi,** dog grass, buchu, corn silk, hydrangea root, and juniper berries.

DOSAGE INFORMATION: The manufacturer suggests taking 2 to 3 tablets with 8 ounces water 2 times a day, 30 minutes before exercise and bedtime.

PRODUCT CLAIMS: Claims are that this product provides the "highest level of L-carnitine in any definition product on the market." It is also described as a leader in nutritional support for weight management and a "serious formula" for people who want a defined physique. The high levels of L-carnitine (converts stored fat into energy), lecithin (helps disperse fats in the body fluids), and inositol (metabolizes fat and combines with choline to form lecithin) appear to support these claims. The proprietary blend provides a diuretic effect.

COMMENTS: If you take this product as directed, the dosage of **L-carnitine** is greater than that recommended as effective, and side effects may occur. If you have diabetes and are taking insulin or any antidiabetic medications, consult your physician before taking this or any product that contains chromium. Chromium has the ability to lower insulin resistance, alter the type or amount of medication needed to control diabetes, and change the frequency with which blood-sugar monitoring should be done.

FURTHER INFORMATION: **Web site:** See www.natrol.com.

Dianixx, by Pharma Botanixx

ACTION: Balances appetite, stops cravings, and helps you feel full.

HOW SOLD: Tablets.

INGREDIENTS: This is a traditional Chinese medicine formula. The blend is proprietary: poria cocos sclerotium (hoelen), plantain, gentiana, rhubarb, cassia seed, chih-shih, prunella, phoenix-tail fern, hsiang-ju, schizandrae fructus, mentha, and licorice.

DOSAGE INFORMATION: The manufacturer suggests taking 3 to 4 tablets 1 hour before meals. Once results have been reached, the instructions are to take 3 to 6 tablets in the morning or afternoon for maintenance.

PRODUCT CLAIMS: The ingredients are said to work synergistically to balance the appetite and stop fat and carbohydrate cravings. They also assist with digestion and help eliminate excess fluid from the body. Hoelen, plantain, prunella, phoenix-tail fern, and hsiang-ju are diuretics. Hoelen also reduces cravings for fats and sugars, and chih-shih makes you feel full very soon after you begin to eat. Rhubarb makes the digestive process begin sooner, and gentiana and chih-shih aid digestion. The manufacturer notes that all the ingredients are 100 percent natural, that no stimulants are used, and that there are no contraindications for use along with over-the-counter drugs.

COMMENTS: The traditional Chinese medicine approach is to treat the whole body; thus, the ingredients in this formula address both symptoms and the underlying problems associated with being overweight. Although this product does not appear to contain any harmful ingredients, its weight-reduction abilities have not been proven.

FURTHER INFORMATION: **Web site:** See Pharma Botanixx at www. strenixx.com.

Diet Fuel, by Twinlab

ACTION: Stimulates metabolism.
HOW SOLD: Capsules.
INGREDIENTS: Three capsules contain: **ephedra**, 334 mg; **guarana** (standardized for 22 percent caffeine), 909 mg; **chromium picolinate**, 200 mcg; **L-carnitine**, 100 mg; HCA, 500 mg; potassium and magnesium phosphate, 100 mg. Also contains bioflavonoids, gingerroot, **green-tea** powder, and **cayenne**. Other ingredients include gelatin, cellulose, purified water, **MCT**, magnesium stearate, and silica.

DOSAGE INFORMATION: The manufacturer recommends that you begin with 1 capsule 3 times a day, one before each meal, to assess your tolerance, and then gradually increase to 3 capsules before each meal. Diet Fuel is to be used as part of a low-fat diet and an exercise program. Instructions remind users to *not* exceed 9 capsules per day.

PRODUCT CLAIMS: Diet Fuel speeds up the metabolism (ephedra, guarana) and helps with the conversion of fats (HCA and chromium). L-carnitine converts stored fats into energy.

COMMENTS: This product contains **ephedra**, which has been linked with serious side effects, including death. It also contains a caffeine-containing substance, **guarana**. This combination is likely to cause anxiety, insomnia, agitation, and other reactions. See individual entries in Part II for warnings. If you have diabetes and are taking insulin or any antidiabetic medications, consult your physician before taking this or any product that contains chromium. Chromium has the ability to lower insulin resistance, alter the type or amount of medication needed to control diabetes, and change the frequency with which blood-sugar monitoring should be done.

Diet Fuel should not be taken by anyone who is pregnant or breast-feeding, or by anyone who is at risk or taking medication for heart disease; high blood pressure; liver or thyroid disease; psychiatric disorders; diabetes; pernicious anemia; nervousness; anxiety; depression; seizure disorders; stroke; or enlarged prostate. Not for use in people younger than eighteen years of age. If you experience dizziness, sleeplessness, headache, tremors, tingling, heart palpitations, or nervousness when taking Diet Fuel, discontinue the product and contact your physician.

FURTHER INFORMATION: **Web site:** See www.twinlab.com.

Diet Therapy, by Polyionics Inc

ACTION: Boosts metabolism.
HOW SOLD: Tablets.

INGREDIENTS: Each tablet contains: citrin (**garcinia cambogia,** minimum 50 percent HCA) 500 mg; **chromium picolinate,** 200 mcg; vanadium, 2 mg; and vitamin B$_3$, 20 mg.

DOSAGE INFORMATION: Package instructions advise taking 1 tablet 30 to 60 minutes before each meal.

PRODUCT CLAIMS: The literature explains that the body combines the vitamin B$_3$ in Diet Therapy with the chromium to make chromium GTF, the form that the body needs to regulate sugar and its storage. The citrin (garcinia cambogia) suppresses appetite, and vanadium supposedly helps control food cravings. The manufacturer notes that Diet Therapy works best when taken with 500 mg L-carnitine. Polyionics recommends one of its own brands, Liqui Carni-B™, but any L-carnitine will suffice.

COMMENTS: There is no reliable scientific evidence to support the manufacturer's claims. If you have diabetes and are taking insulin or any antidiabetic medications, consult your physician before taking this or any product that contains chromium. Chromium has the ability to lower insulin resistance, alter the type or amount of medication needed to control diabetes, and change the frequency with which blood-sugar monitoring should be done.

FURTHER INFORMATION: **Web site:** See www.nutritionfarm.com.

Diurlean, by ISS Research

ACTION: A combination of metabolic stimulants, lipotropic agents, and herbal diuretics.

HOW SOLD: Capsules.

INGREDIENTS: Three capsules (1 dose) contain the following: ma huang (**ephedra**), 300 mg; **guarana**, 150 mg; caffeine, 80 mg; **citrus aurantium**, 200 mg; white willow, 100 mg; tyrosine, 100 mg; vitamin B$_5$, 10 mg; choline bitartrate, 250 mg; inositol, 250 mg; betaine hydrochloride, 100 mg; **carnitine** L-tartarate, 50 mg; lipase, 200 LU; **chromium** chelavite, 300 mcg. There is also a list of herbs in a proprietary powder blend (500 mg); these include alfalfa; bladderwrack, **cayenne** pepper; corn silk; **dandelion**; gingerroot; **kelp**; marshmallow root; **parsley**; and peppermint.

DOSAGE INFORMATION: According to the manufacturer, take 3 capsules 1 to 2 times per day with meals.

PRODUCT CLAIMS: Claims are that this product will stimulate and increase your body's ability to burn fat and calories. Of the primary ingredients, ma huang (**ephedra**), **guarana**, and caffeine stimulate metabolism; inositol combines with choline to form lecithin, which helps disperse fats in body fluids. The proprietary blend contains both diuretics and metabolic stimulants. For best results, the labeling suggests that consumers use this product along with a low-fat diet and exercise.

COMMENTS: Diurlean™ contains **ephedra**, which has been linked with serious side effects, including death. It also contains a caffeine-containing substance, **guarana**, as well as caffeine. This combination is likely to cause anxiety, insomnia, agitation, and other reactions. See individual entries in Part II for details.

FURTHER INFORMATION: **Web site:** See www.issresearch.com.

Dr. Art Ulene's Weight Loss Kit

ACTION: 28-day weight loss kit.

HOW SOLD: The kit contains CarboBurner capsules, Herbal-Energizer tablets, and NutritionBoost vitamins, all of which are considered to be one packet. The kit also includes a dietary guide and progress chart.

INGREDIENTS: Each packet contains the following: vitamin A (50 percent as beta-carotene), 1,667 IU; vitamin C, 60 mg; vitamin D, 133 IU; vitamin E (as d-alpha tocopherol, 20 IU; vitamin K, 27 mcg; thiamine (B_1), 10.5 mg; riboflavin (B_2), 0.6 mg; niacinamide (B_3), 6.7 mg; pyridoxine (B_6), 1.3 mg; folic acid, 133 mcg; vitamin B_{12}, 33 mcg; biotin, 33 mcg; pantothenic acid (B_5), 3.3 mg; calcium (carbonate), 100 mg; iron (ferrus fumarate), 2.7 mg; iodine, 33 mcg; magnesium, 103 mg; selenium, 67 mcg; copper, 1 mg; manganese, 0.7 mg; **chromium** (polynicotinate and picolinate), 240 mcg; molybdenum, 25 mcg; **ginseng** (Korean), 100 mg; citrus bioflavonoids, 17 mg; boron, 0.3 mg; vanadium, 300 mcg. Also contains microcrystalline cellulose; di-calcium phosphate; dextrose; calcium carbonate; stearic acid; croscamellose sodium; gelatin; starch; magnesium stearate; vanillin; sodium starch glycolate; dextrin; lecithin; sodium carboxymethylcellulose; FD&C yellow No. 6 lake; polyethylene glycol 8000NF; titanium dioxide; sodium citrate; FD&C red No. 40 lake; FD&C blue No. 2 lake.

DOSAGE INFORMATION: The manufacturer's directions advise users to follow the Step-by-Step Guide and Progress Chart and to take 1 packet 3 times a day with meals.

PRODUCT CLAIMS: The CarboBurner capsules (vanadium, chromium, and thiamine) help the body transform carbohydrates into energy instead of fat. The HerbalEnergizer tablets contain ginseng, which helps increase your energy level. The vitamin-mineral mixture enhances your daily dietary intake. The manufacturer claims that when these products are taken with food, they will perform these functions in an optimal fashion.

COMMENTS: This product provides a well-balanced nutritional supplement program to accompany a reduced-calorie diet and exercise program. However, there are no reliable scientific studies to support the claims that CarboBurner and Herbal-Engerizer supplements will enhance weight loss. If you have diabetes and are taking insulin or any antidiabetic medications, consult your physician before taking this or any product that contains chromium. Chromium has the ability to lower insulin resistance, alter the type or amount of medication needed to control diabetes, and change the frequency with which blood-sugar monitoring should be done.

This weight-loss program was devised by Dr. Art Ulene, a clinical professor at the University of Southern California School of Medicine. He has authored more than fifty books, videos, and audiotapes on health topics.

FURTHER INFORMATION: Contact/Web site: If you have questions about this product, you can call Dr. Art Ulene's Nutritional and Product Information Hotline at 1-800-DR-ULENE; www.DrArtUlene.com.

Dr. Art Ulene's CarboBurner

ACTION: Stimulates metabolism.

HOW SOLD: Capsules.

INGREDIENTS: Each capsule contains thiamine (vitamin B_1), 10 mg; magnesium, 35 mg; **chromium**, 200 mcg; vanadium, 300 mcg. Other ingredients include: powdered cellulose; gelatin; magnesium stearate; sodium starch glycolate; pregelatinized starch.

DOSAGE INFORMATION: A typical dosage is 3 capsules per day, one with each meal.

PRODUCT CLAIMS: When taken with food, this product supports the body's ability to convert carbohydrates into energy instead of fat.

COMMENTS: If you have diabetes and are taking insulin or any antidiabetic medications, consult your physician before taking this or any product that contains chromium. Chromium has the ability to lower insulin resistance, alter the type or amount of medication needed to control diabetes, and change the frequency with which blood-sugar monitoring should be done.

This product was devised by Dr. Art Ulene, a clinical professor at the University of Southern California School of Medicine. He has authored more than fifty books, videos, and audiotapes on health topics.

FURTHER INFORMATION: **Contact/Web site:** If you have questions about this product, you can call Dr. Art Ulene's Nutritional and Product Information Hotline at 1-800-DR-ULENE; www.DrArtUlene.com.

Dr. Duncan's Diet & Cleansing Plan, by Nature's Secret

ACTION: Promotes weight loss and internal body cleansing.

HOW SOLD: Tablets.

INGREDIENTS: Two tablets contain the following: **psyllium** seed husk, 200 mg; **uva ursi** leaf, 200 mg; **cascara sagrada**, 110 mg; juniper berry, 100 mg; prune powder, 90 mg; grapefruit powder, 80 mg; beet root powder, 80 mg; oat fiber, 80 mg; **chick-weed** powder, 50 mg; **dandelion** root powder, 50 mg; chlorella (a green alga), 50 mg; echinacea, 40 mg; gingerroot, 40 mg; chamomile extract, 25 mg; fenugreek extract, 25 mg. Also contains a proprietary blend (100 mg) of fennel seed; marshmallow-root extract; casanthranol bark; FOS; **cayenne**; and Bioperine. Other ingredients include microcrystalline; cellulose; stearic acid; croscarmellose sodium; and magnesium stearate. The product is free of yeast, wheat, corn, dairy, and artificial colors, flavors, and preservatives.

DOSAGE INFORMATION: A Cleansing Diet booklet comes with the product and advises taking 2 tablets 3 times a day for 7 days, then taking 2 tablets 2 times a day as a maintenance dose. Drink 8 to 10 glasses of water daily.

PRODUCT CLAIMS: The literature claims that this is a "revolutionary formula" that eliminates toxins from the body and promotes healthy weight loss. The primary ingredients responsible for this action are chlorella, which energizes the body; and juniper berry, uva ursi, cascara, and psyllium, which help with internal cleansing through urination and stool elimination.

This formula was designed by Lindsey Duncan, N.D., C.N., who chose specific "harmonizing" herbs and botanicals. The literature notes that "many of the herbs in this formula have been used for centuries by cultures around the world and cannot be found in other formulas."

COMMENTS: Dr. Duncan's Diet & Cleansing Plan contains the very potent laxative **cascara sagrada**, which should not be taken along with other laxatives. Yet the plan also contains several other laxatives in the form of oat fiber and several vegetable and fruit fibers, which may increase the possibility for serious side effects. See Part II for details.

Do not take this product if you have diarrhea, loose stools, or abdominal pain; or if you are pregnant, breast-feeding, taking medication, or have a medical condition.

FURTHER INFORMATION: **Web site**: See www.naturessecret.com.

Elim Slim, by Gaia Herbs

ACTION: Advertised as an aid for weight balance.

HOW SOLD: Liquid extract.

INGREDIENTS: Green-tea leaf; garcinia-malabar tamarind (**garcinia cambogia**); coleus forskohlii root; elderberry berry; **gymnema sylvestre** leaf; bladderwrack (**kelp**) fronds; licorice root; jujube date seed; turmeric root; fresh gingerroot; pure grain alcohol (40 to 50 percent); and spring water.

DOSAGE INFORMATION: The manufacturer suggests taking 40 to 60 drops in a small amount of warm water 3 to 4 times a day between meals.

PRODUCT CLAIMS: The green tea and bladderwrack stimulate metabolism; the garcinia cambogia suppresses appetite; and licorice and gingerroot aid digestion.

Elim Slim is a certified organic extract. The manufacturer recommends that you consult a professional nutritionist or other person knowledgeable about nutrition for advice on how to use this product for weight balance.

COMMENTS: The exact amount of each ingredient is unknown; therefore, you cannot know whether this product contains any substance in an amount reportedly sufficient to assist in weight loss. Do not use Elim Slim if you are pregnant or breast-feeding.

FURTHER INFORMATION: **Web site:** See www.gaiaherbs.com.

Enforma System: Exercise in a Bottle and Fat Trapper, by Enforma

ACTION: Burns fat, eliminates fat.

HOW SOLD: Two products used together: both capsules.

INGREDIENTS: Exercise in a Bottle consists of **pyruvate**; ginkgo; **chromium picolinate**; and **garcinia cambogia**. Fat Trapper contains **chitosan** and **psyllium** husk (marketed as Chitozyme™).

DOSAGE INFORMATION: Fat Trapper: The manufacturer suggests taking 1 to 5 capsules 30 to 60 minutes before each high-fat meal. For Exercise in a Bottle: Instructions are to take at least

1 capsule per day, or take 1 in the morning and 1 in early afternoon.

PRODUCT CLAIMS: The manufacturer claims that Fat Trapper surrounds the fat in the foods that you eat and binds the fat together so that it cannot be absorbed by the body. It is then eliminated in the stool. The pyruvate in Exercise in a Bottle stimulates metabolism while garcinia cambogia suppresses appetite, chromium picolinate suppresses cravings, and ginkgo helps the cells function more efficiently. The Enforma System comes with a twenty-four-page booklet on diet and exercise that should be followed if you want to see results.

The Enforma System is advertised as being for people with busy lifestyles. The product claims to increase the activity of muscle cells, enabling them to burn stored fat.

COMMENTS: The Federal Trade Commission (FTC) settled a $10 million law suit with Enforma in 2000 over false advertising claims made by the manufacturer about Fat Trapper. As a result of the settlement, Enforma can no longer say that its chitosan product (1) prevents the absorption of fat in the human body; (2) enables people to lose weight without having to exercise; and (3) enables people to lose weight and continue to eat high-fat foods. For more information about this case, see Further Information.

If you have diabetes and are taking insulin or any antidiabetic medications, consult your physician before taking this or any product that contains chromium. Chromium has the ability to lower insulin resistance, alter the type or amount of medication needed to control diabetes, and change the frequency with which blood-sugar monitoring should be done. Before taking this product, consult your doctor if you are pregnant or breast-feeding, taking medication, or if you have heart disease or high blood pressure. The manufacturer reports that there are no side effects from use of this product.

FURTHER INFORMATION: **Web site:** See www.skepticfriends.org and http://webmd.lycos.com/content/article/1728.54465.

Fat Burner, by California Health

ACTION: Stimulates metabolism.

HOW SOLD: Capsules.

INGREDIENTS: Two capsules contain: thiamine (vitamin B_1), 25 mg; riboflavin (vitamin B_2), 25 mg; niacinamide, 25 mg; **chromium** (amino-acid chelate), 200 mcg; alpha-lipoic acid, 200 mcg; **pyruvate** (as calcium and potassium), 800 mg. Inactive ingredients include gelatin; cellulose; calcium phosphate hydrous; magnesium stearate.

DOSAGE INFORMATION: Package instructions advise taking 2 to 6 capsules per day along with a low-calorie diet and exercise.

PRODUCT CLAIMS: The manufacturer claims that the pyruvate in Fat Burner increases cellular respiration (the use of energy) and the amount of fat used as energy. It can slightly increase the rate of metabolism, which in turn enhances the burning of fat. The addition of calcium and potassium helps the pyruvate digest properly in the intestines. Chromium helps control blood-sugar levels and is involved in the metabolism of fat, protein, and carbohydrates.

COMMENTS: No research is offered to back up the claims made by the manufacturer. If you have diabetes and are taking insulin or any antidiabetic medications, consult your physician before taking this or any product that contains chromium. Chromium has the ability to lower insulin resistance, alter the type or amount of medication needed to control diabetes, and change the frequency with which blood-sugar monitoring should be done.

FURTHER INFORMATION: **Contact/Web site:** California Health, E-mail for information: info@calhealth.com; www.calhealth.com.

Fat Grabbers, by Nature's Sunshine

ACTION: Traps fat; also helps control cholesterol and blood-sugar levels.

HOW SOLD: Capsules.

INGREDIENTS: **Chickweed**; lecithin; **psyllium** husk; **guar gum**.

DOSAGE INFORMATION: A typical dosage is 1 capsule with water before each meal.

PRODUCT CLAIMS: This product is advertised as being one that "assists" with any type of weight-management program. Fat Grabbers reportedly "traps fat molecules" in the intestines before they can make their way to the bloodstream. In fact, the directions suggest that Fat Grabbers be used with a sensible diet plan and exercise in order to be effective.

The manufacturer reports that clinical trials were performed in Norway in which Fat Grabbers was studied in sixty-four overweight and obese individuals. The placebo-controlled, double-blind study lasted 12 weeks and was conducted by Dr. Erling Thom, Ph.D., who works as the head of clinical operations in the Parexel Medstat Region in Nordic countries. The results were not published in a peer-reviewed journal.

The average amount of weight lost by subjects who took Fat Grabbers was 16 pounds, compared with 8 pounds in those who took placebos. In addition to weight loss, total cholesterol levels decreased 0.53 mmol/L in the Fat Grabbers group and 0.38 mmol/L in the placebo group. Fat Grabbers also significantly reduced hunger pangs and did not cause side effects. In addition, the press release from Nature's Sunshine reports that subjects who took Fat Grabbers "experienced an 81% weight reduction due to fat loss, with a minimum loss of water and lean muscle tissue when consuming the product three times per day complemented with light exercise and a low-fat diet." The manufacturer reports that additional studies to determine the long-term benefits, safety, and tolerability of Fat Grabbers are underway.

COMMENTS: The amount of each ingredient in this product is unknown. Grabbers is basically a laxative with questionable fat-dissolving abilities. Unbiased peer-reviewed research is needed to identify whether Fat Grabbers is an effective weight-loss aid.

FURTHER INFORMATION: **Web site:** See www.healthy-sunshine.com.

Glucomannan+, by Swanson

ACTION: Suppresses appetite.

HOW SOLD: Capsules.

INGREDIENTS: Two capsules contain: **psyllium** husk fiber, 600 mg; konjac **glucomannan**, 450 mg; apple pectin, 300 mg; **chitosan** (93 percent deacetylated), 300 mg; **guar gum**, 300 mg; oat bran fiber, 300 mg; **chromium** (50 percent from Chromax chromium picolinate, 50 percent from chromium polynicolinate), 150 mcg; **gymnema sylvestre** extract (25 percent gymnemic acids), 75 mg; **L-carnitine** (as L-carnitine tartrate), 30 mg.

DOSAGE INFORMATION: Package directions advise taking 2 to 3 capsules 3 times per day with water.

PRODUCT CLAIMS: The psyllium, glucomannan, apple pectin, guar gum, and oat bran create a feeling of fullness; the chromium and gymnema reduce cravings for sugar and carbohydrates; and chitosan absorbs fat.

COMMENTS: The fiber ingredients—psyllium, glucomannan, apple pectin, guar gum, and oat bran—likely work well as a laxative, but only if you drink at least 64 ounces of water daily when taking this product in order to promote elimination of the fiber. Using laxatives, however, is not an effective or safe way to lose weight. Chitosan has been shown to be an *ineffective* product.

If you have diabetes and are taking insulin or any antidiabetic medications, consult your physician before taking this or any product that contains chromium. Chromium has the ability to lower insulin resistance, alter the type or amount of medication needed to control diabetes, and change the frequency with which blood-sugar monitoring should be done.

FURTHER INFORMATION: This product is available by mail order and via Internet: www.swansonvitamins.com.

Grapefruit 60, The Fat-Burner Diet Plan; Grapefruit Fat Burner Diet with Niacin, both by Head Start

ACTION: Burns fat.

HOW SOLD: Tablets.

INGREDIENTS: 100 percent pure grapefruit extract in a base of tri-calcium phosphate (230 mg); citrus bioflavonoids (10 mg); and grapefruit pectin (10 mg). The Niacin formula also contains vitamin B_3, which is used to control cholesterol. However, cholesterol lowering requires much higher doses of B_3 than this product produces (see below).

DOSAGE INFORMATION: The plan booklet included with Grapefruit 60 explains how to use the tablets along with a diet plan.

PRODUCT CLAIMS: The manufacturer emphasizes that its Fat Burner Diet Plan includes "some very sensible suggestions" about the types of foods users of Grapefruit 60 should consume if they want to take advantage of the "synergistic metabolism" that will speed up weight loss safely and naturally. The plan booklet instructs users to keep calorie intake between 800 and 1,200 calories per day for best results. The addition of niacin to the second formulation is meant to lower cholesterol. However, the manufacturer states that each tablet contains only 7 mg of niacin, whereas the dose used to lower cholesterol is up to 3,000 mg.

Proof of the effectiveness of this product is offered by the manufacturer, who notes that a University of Florida researcher, Dr. James Cerda, found that pectin derived from grapefruit rinds has a dramatic cholesterol-lowering effect on the arteries of pigs fed a high-fat diet. This study has not been done in humans, however.

COMMENTS: This product is another variation of the grapefruit diet that has been circulating for decades. There is no scientific basis for this weight-loss plan.

FURTHER INFORMATION: **Web site:** www.headstartvitamins.com.

Greens Today Fat Burning, by Organic Frog

ACTION: Promotes burning of fat.

HOW SOLD: Capsules.

INGREDIENTS: The capsules are in a base of tomato powder; tangerine bioflavonoid; cherry juice powder; broccoli powder; kale powder; and carrot powder. Each 12 capsules contain: **garcinia**

cambogia, 2,000 mg; tyrosine, 500 mg; **guggulipid** extract (**guggul**), 500 mg; **spirulina,** 350 mg; soy lecithin (95 percent phosphatides), 350 mg; apple fiber, 250 mg; **L-carnitine,** 250 mg; triphala extract, 250 mg; methionine, 250 mg; borage powder, 200 mg; **uva ursi,** 200 mg; bladderwrack (**kelp**), 200 mg; Jerusalem artichoke powder, 187.5 mg; fenugreek, 150 mg; chlorella, 150 mg; **cascara sagrada,** 150 mg; glycine, 125 mg; lysine, 125 mg; calcium (carbonate, citrate, and maleate), 125 mg; watercress, 100 mg; potassium citrate, 94 mg; alfalfa juice powder, 87.5 mg; barley juice powder, 87.5 mg; wheat grass juice powder, 87.5 mg; carob, 87.5 mg; brown rice bran, 87.5 mg; flaxseed meal, 87.5 mg; FOS, 75 mg; vitamin C, 62.5 mg; dairy-free lactobacillus acidophilus, 62.5 mL; *L. bulgaricus,* 62.5 mL; *L. coagulans,* 62.5 mL; *Bifidobacterium bifidus,* 62.5 mL; wild yam, 60 mg; **cayenne,** 50 mg; barberry, 50 mg; vitamin A (beta-carotene), 1,250 IU; vitamin D, 100 IU; vitamin E (natural), 50 IU; acerola berry juice powder, 37.5 mg; red beet juice powder, 31.5 mg; wild imported rose hips, 31.5 mg; bromelain, 25 mg; licorice root powder, 25 mg; spinach powder, 25 mg; oat bran concentrate, 25 mg; **Siberian ginseng,** 20 mg; plant-based digestive enzymes, 19 mg; vitamin B_{12}, 6.5 mcg; **astragalus membranaceus,** 12.5 mg; royal jelly, 12.5 mg; cholestatin, 12.5 mg; phosphorus, 12.5 mg; Bioperine, 10 mg; pau d'arco powder, 9 mg; fo-ti powder, 9 mg; red dulse powder, 9 mg; milk thistle (standardized extract 80 percent), 9 mg; **dandelion** root powder, 9 mg; hawthorn berry (standardized extract 4:1), 9 mg; Spanish bee pollen, 6.5 mg; gingerroot powder, 6.5 mg; burdock root powder, 6.5 mg; reishi mushroom, 6.5 mg; echinacea (standardized extract), 6.5 mg; slippery elm bark, 6.5 mg; silica, 6.25 mg; niacin, 5 mg; zinc, 4 mg; alpha-lipoic acid, 2.5 mg; **maitake** mushroom, 2.5 mg; ginkgo biloba, 2.5 mg; shiitake mushroom, 2.5 mg; grapeseed (standardized extract 90 percent), 2.5 mg; pycnogenol, 2.5 mg; Japanese **green tea,** 2.5 mg; Norwegian sea **kelp,** 2.5 mg; bilberry, 2.5 mg; horsetail, 2.5 mg; vitamin B_5, 2.5 mg; vitamin B_6, 1.5 mg; vitamin B_1 (thiamine), 1 mg; iron, 1 mg; vitamin B_2 (riboflavin), 0.5 mg; copper gluconate, 0.5 mg; manganese, 0.5 mg; boron (citrate and gluconate), 0.5 mg;

vitamin B_3, 0.5 mg; Co-Q10, 250 mcg; octocosanol, 250 mcg; folic acid, 100 mcg; biotin, 75 mcg; magnesium citrate, 62.5 mcg; **chromium picolinate,** 62.5 mcg; iodine (kelp), 37.5 mcg; molybdenum, 19 mcg; selenium, 17.5 mcg; vanadium, 12.5 mcg.

DOSAGE INFORMATION: According to the manufacturer, the typical dosage is four capsules 30 to 60 minutes before each meal.

PRODUCT CLAIMS: This product contains a wide variety of nutrients and herbals that may support the body during dieting. The high dose of garcinia cambogia is supposed to prevent carbohydrates from transforming into fats and suppresses appetite.

COMMENTS: There are no scientific studies to support the claims made about **garcinia cambogia**. The very potent **cascara sagrada** is present, but not in an alarming dosage. As for the remaining ingredients, the majority may provide sound nutritional support for individuals who are dieting, but there is no scientific evidence that they promote weight loss.

Greens Today contains no dairy; wheat; corn; animal products; artificial colors or flavors; synthetic chemicals or preservatives; MSG; lactose; sucrose; fructose; dextrose; egg; yeast; or added salt. Individuals who are allergic to bee pollen should note that this product contains it.

FURTHER INFORMATION: **Contact:** 1-800-GREEN41; **Web site:** www.organicfrog.com.

Herbal Diet Max, by NaturalMax

ACTION: Controls appetite, burns fat.

HOW SOLD: Capsules.

INGREDIENTS: One capsule contains ma huang, 400 mg (4 mg [1 percent] **ephedra** alkaloids minimum); bitter orange (**citrus aurantium** guaranteed 15 mg [6 percent] synephrine), 250 mg; **green-tea** extract, 200 mg; white willow, 50 mg. Also contains gelatin; cellulose; ginger; **cayenne**; cinnamon; black pepper; and magnesium stearate.

DOSAGE INFORMATION: A typical dosage is 1 capsule in the morning and 1 in early afternoon.

PRODUCT CLAIMS: The four primary ingredients, plus the cayenne and ginger, all stimulate metabolism. The product comes with the NaturalMax Diet Plan, which emphasizes sensible eating and exercise in order to achieve weight loss.

COMMENTS: This product contains **ephedra**, which has been linked with serious side effects, including death. See individual entry for **ephedra** in Part II, pp. 67–70.

Consult your doctor before taking Herbal Diet Max if you are pregnant or breast-feeding; if you have high blood pressure; heart or thyroid disease; glaucoma; diabetes; an enlarged prostate; or are taking MAO inhibitors or any other prescription medication. Stop taking the product if you experience nervousness, nausea, or sleeplessness. Excessive or improper use of the product can cause rapid heartbeat and nervousness and may be hazardous to your health. This product is not for individuals younger than eighteen years of age. Citrus aurantium may cause sensitivity to UV (ultraviolet) exposure.

FURTHER INFORMATION: **Web site:** See www.nutraceutical.com.

Herbal Phen-Fen, by HPF LLC

ACTION: Suppresses appetite.

HOW SOLD: Tablets.

INGREDIENTS: Two tablets contain 650 mg of a proprietary formula: St. John's wort (standardized 0.3 percent hypericin), ma huang (**ephedra**) extract (standardized 8 percent alkaloids); also dicalcium phosphate; microcrystalline cellulose; croscarmellose sodium; stearic acid; silica; magnesium stearate; and pharmaceutical glaze.

DOSAGE INFORMATION: The manufacturer suggests 2 tablets, 2 to 3 times daily, 30 minutes before meals.

PRODUCT CLAIMS: St. John's wort prolongs the reuptake of the neurotransmitter serotonin in the brain. Serotonin reduces appetite and helps you feel full. Ma huang increases the metabolism rate and helps control hunger. The manufacturer notes that when HPH Herbal Phen-Fen is combined with a low-calorie diet and exercise, it can help you lose weight.

The manufacturer reports on a study conducted at St. Lukes–Roosevelt Memorial Hospital in New York City in which ma huang and St. John's wort were given to obese individuals in an open-label trial. During an 8-week period, more than 800 subjects received 40 mg ma huang and 800 mg St. John's wort daily. At 4 weeks, the subjects had lost a mean of 1.72 pounds per week; at 8 weeks, the mean weight loss was 1.4 pounds per week. COMMENTS: HPF Herbal Phen-Fen is a proprietary blend that was created as a nonprescription alternative to the now-unavailable prescription Phen-Fen. It contains **ephedra**, which has been linked with serious side effects, including death. See individual entry for **ephedra** (pp. 67–70) in Part II for details.

Use of HPF Herbal Phen-Fen is not recommended if you are pregnant, breast-feeding, or taking an MAO inhibitor. If you have diabetes, prostate enlargement, heart disease, thyroid disease, or high blood pressure, consult your doctor before taking this product.

FURTHER INFORMATION: **Contact:** Open-label weight-loss trial of combination herbal ma huang and St. John's wort. Steven B. Heymsfield, Obesity Research Center, St. Lukes–Roosevelt Memorial Hospital, Columbia University, New York, NY 10025.

Herbal Phen Fuel Plus, by Twinlab

ACTION: Stimulates metabolism.

HOW SOLD: Capsules.

INGREDIENTS: Two capsules contain **citrus aurantium**, 325 mg; St. John's wort (standardized 0.3 percent hypericin), 300 mg; **L-phenylalanine**, 50 mg; **guarana**, 800 mg. The product is in an herbal, thermogenic base of coleus forskohlii extract; **green-tea** powder; citrus bioflavonoids (containing naringin); gingerroot powder; **cayenne** powder; and yohimbine bark extract. It does not contain sugar, salt, or artificial colors, flavors, or preservatives.

DOSAGE INFORMATION: The manufacturer says to take 2 capsules with water before each meal and not to exceed 6 capsules per day.

PRODUCT CLAIMS: The manufacturer claims that it can lead to weight loss when used as part of a calorie-controlled diet and exercise plan.

COMMENTS: This product contains a large amount of the caffeine-containing substance **guarana**, which can cause significant side effects (see entry in Part II, pp. 82–84, for details). Do not use this product if you are pregnant, breast-feeding, or if you have or are at risk for high blood pressure; heart, liver, or thyroid disease; psychiatric disorders; diabetes; pernicious anemia; nervousness; anxiety; depression; seizure disorders; stroke; or an enlarged prostate. Consult your doctor if you are taking MAO inhibitors or any other prescription drugs before taking Herbal Phen Fuel Plus. This product is not for people younger than eighteen years of age. Discontinue use if you experience dizziness, headache, heart palpitations, or tingling.

FURTHER INFORMATION: **Web site:** See www.twinlab.com.

Herbazings, by Ageless Company

ACTION: Detoxifies and promotes urination.

HOW SOLD: Capsules (gelatin).

INGREDIENTS: Each 500-mg capsule contains a proprietary blend of parsley, basil, celery, and fennel.

DOSAGE INFORMATION: The manufacturer advises taking 1 to 2 capsules per day with lots of water, about two 8-ounce glasses.

PRODUCT CLAIMS: Herbazings are designed to flush the kidneys, assist with weight loss, and detoxify the body by getting rid of toxins that accumulate while you diet.

COMMENTS: All of the ingredients in Herbazings have been used by herbalists, many for centuries, as detoxifiers. Parsley flushes the kidneys and is a mild laxative; basil helps the digestive process and relieves depression; celery relieves stress; and fennel enhances metabolism. The product may be helpful as a detoxifier while you are dieting, but do not expect it to be useful as a weight-loss aid.

FURTHER INFORMATION: **Web site:** www.ageless.com.za.

Medi-Thin Day, by Nature's Gold

ACTION: Stimulates metabolism.

HOW SOLD: Caplets.

INGREDIENTS: Each caplet contains **ephedra**, 150 mg; **guarana** extract, 90 mg; **kola nut** extract, 90 mg; **garcinia cambogia**, 60 mg; white willow bark, 50 mg; **Siberian ginseng** extract, 50 mg; bladderwrack (**kelp**) extract, 50 mg; licorice root, 50 mg; St. John's wort, 15 mg; chromium chelate and **chromium picolinate**, 400 mcg; **L-carnitine**; and **green-tea** extract.

DOSAGE INFORMATION: Information not provided by manufacturer.

PRODUCT CLAIMS: The ephedra, guarana, kola nut, white willow bark, ginseng, and bladderwrack stimulate the metabolism; garcinia suppresses the appetite; St. Johns wort is a mild sedative and appetite suppressant; chromium reduces sugar and carbohydrate cravings; licorice aids digestion; L-carnitine helps convert stored fat into energy; and green tea is a diuretic and a metabolic stimulator.

COMMENTS: This product contains **ephedra**, which has been linked with serious side effects, including death. It also contains two caffeine-containing substances, **guarana** and **kola nut**. This three-herb combination is likely to cause anxiety, insomnia, agitation, and other adverse reactions.

This product should not be taken by people younger than eighteen, pregnant or breast-feeding women, or anyone who has a medical condition. If you have diabetes and are taking insulin or any antidiabetic medications, consult with your physician before taking this or any product that contains chromium. Chromium has the ability to lower insulin resistance, alter the type or amount of medication needed to control diabetes, and change the frequency with which blood-sugar monitoring should be done.

FURTHER INFORMATION: **Web site:** See www.naturesgold.com.

Metabolic Thyrolean, by ProLab

ACTION: Influences metabolism.

HOW SOLD: Capsules.

INGREDIENTS: Six capsules contain the following: calcium phosphate, 750 mg; dipotassium phosphate, 450 mg; L-tyrosine, 750 mg; **garcinia cambogia**, 750 mg; gum **guggul** extract, 750 mg; sodium phosphate, 225 mg; disodium phosphate, 225 mg; phosphatidylcholine (lecithin), 75 mg.

DOSAGE INFORMATION: Per the manufacturer's instructions, Metabolic Thyrolean should be taken before meals using the following schedule: 2 capsules (1 before each of 2 meals) on days 1 through 3; increase to 4 capsules on days 4 through 7; then increase again to 6 capsules after day 7, with the result being 2 capsules 3 times daily with meals.

PRODUCT CLAIMS: Advertisements for Metabolic Thyrolean claim that it operates on the principle that when people go on a diet, their thyroid hormone levels, metabolic rate, and certain neurotransmitter levels decline. These factors can cause weight loss to stop. Metabolic Thyrolean tackles healthy weight loss by providing nutrients that preserve or increase thyroid output (the thyroid gland controls metabolism), preserve or increase metabolic rate, and promote production of neurotransmitters (epinephrine and norepinephrine).

COMMENTS: The claims that Metabolic Thyrolean can increase healthy fat loss when used alone and may help herbal fat burners work more efficiently are not supported by reliable scientific studies.

If you are pregnant, breast-feeding, younger than eighteen years of age, or taking MAO inhibitors, consult your doctor before taking this product.

FURTHER INFORMATION: **Web site:** www.prolab.com.

Metabolife 356

ACTION: Stimulates metabolism.

HOW SOLD: Caplets.

INGREDIENTS: Each caplet contains: vitamin E, 6 IU; magnesium, 75 mg; zinc, 5 mg; **chromium picolinate**, 75 mcg. The proprietary blend (728 mg) includes **guarana** (40 mg naturally occurring caffeine); **ephedra** (12 mg naturally occurring ephedrines); bee pollen; **ginseng** root; gingerroot; lecithin; bovine complex; damiana leaf; sarsaparilla root; goldenseal; nettles leaf; gotu kola; and **spirulina**. Inert ingredients include methocel; silica; croscarmellose; sodium; and magnesium stearate.

DOSAGE INFORMATION: Package instructions advise taking 2 to 3 servings per day at least 4 hours apart and no more than 1 hour before a meal. A serving is determined according to body weight. The directions suggest taking 1 caplet and for each 30 pounds over 120 pounds, adding ½ caplet. The manufacturer recommends not exceeding 2 caplets per serving or 8 caplets per day. Within 1 hour of taking a dose, a decrease in appetite and an increase in energy level may occur, according to the manufacturer. Each caplet should be taken with at least 16 ounces of water (e.g., 1½ caplets should be taken with 24 ounces of water). The diuretics in Metabolife 356 require this level of fluid intake.

The morning dose should be taken before a high-protein breakfast. All meals and snacks should include healthy, nutritious foods.

PRODUCT CLAIMS: The literature notes that Metabolife 356 works better when you eat; therefore, skipping meals is discouraged. Eating small meals and light snacks in between is suggested to help maintain a healthy blood-sugar balance and to prevent hunger. The manufacturer claims that Metabolife 356 will increase your metabolic rate, decrease your appetite, and burn fat without the need to diet or exercise.

The literature stresses that weight loss should not exceed 7 to 11 pounds per month. If you lose weight at a faster rate, you are encouraged to reduce your use of Metabolife 356 or increase your food intake.

COMMENTS: This product contains **ephedra**, which has been linked with serious side effects, including death. It also contains a caffeine-containing substance, **guarana**. This combination is likely to cause anxiety, insomnia, agitation, and other reactions. Individuals allergic to bee pollen should note that this product contains an unknown amount.

If you have diabetes and are taking insulin or any anti-diabetic medications, consult with your physician before taking this or any product that contains chromium. Chromium has the ability to lower insulin resistance, alter the type or amount of medication needed to control diabetes, and change the frequency with which blood-sugar monitoring should be done.

If you experience nausea, lightheadedness, gas, or dizziness when taking Metabolife 356, it is suggested that you eat one serving of a low- or no-fat dairy food or soymilk within 10 minutes of taking your dose. If the symptoms subside but do not disappear, reduce your Metabolife 356 dose. If symptoms remain, stop taking Metabolife 356.

Do not take Metabolife 356 if you are pregnant, breast-feeding, or younger than eighteen years; have high blood pressure, diabetes, an enlarged prostate, heart disease, or thyroid disease; or if you are taking an MAO inhibitor or any other prescription medications.

The manufacturer's literature notes that Metabolife 356 has undergone medical safety studies at two independent laboratories and has been tested clinically at two major universities in the United States, although the labs and universities are not named and the results of the studies are not revealed.

FURTHER INFORMATION: **Web site:** See www.metabolife.com.

MetaboTrim™ by Natural Health Company

ACTION: Suppresses appetite, stimulates metabolism.
HOW SOLD: Capsules.
INGREDIENTS: Fully identified ingredients include HCA (**garcinia cambogia**), 500 mg; **chromium picolinate**, 100 mcg; vitamin C, 50 mg; vitamin B_6, 25 mg; and vitamin B_{12}, 25 mg. The proprietary blend includes **DL-phenylalanine**; bee pollen; L-methionine; **L-carnitine**; L-tyrosine; L-proline; dandelion; licorice; **kelp**; bissy nut (**kola nut**); gotu kola; and white willow bark.

DOSAGE INFORMATION: A typical dosage is 4 capsules per day: 2 in the morning and 2 midday, with water.

PRODUCT CLAIMS: The HCA, chromium picolinate, bissy nut (kola nut), and DL-phenylalanine stimulate the metabolism and burn fat; the bissy nut, L-tyrosine, and dandelion suppress the appetite; bee pollen and gotu kola provide energy; L-methionine prevents fat buildup; L-carnitine transforms fat into energy; and white willow bark increases the effects of the other herbs.

COMMENTS: Note that this product contains the DL form of phenylalanine, which is not the form reported to be the most helpful for obesity. If you have diabetes and are taking insulin or any antidiabetic medications, consult with your physician before taking this or any product that contains chromium. Chromium has the ability to lower insulin resistance, alter the type or amount of medication needed to control diabetes, and change the frequency with which blood-sugar monitoring should be done. Individuals who are allergic to bee pollen should note that this product contains an unknown amount of it.

FURTHER INFORMATION: **Web site:** See www.naturalhealthco.com.

Minolest, by Bionax

ACTION: Suppresses appetite.

HOW SOLD: Powder, sold in packets.

INGREDIENTS: **Psyllium, glucomannan,** and **guar gum**.

DOSAGE INFORMATION: The package directions are to mix the contents of a packet with water and drink it immediately, or allow it to sit for about 10 minutes until it turns jellylike and eat it with a spoon. The recommended dosage is 2 to 3 packets per day.

PRODUCT CLAIMS: Minolest provides fiber that makes you feel full and therefore less likely to overeat. Proof of this claim appeared in a study published in the *American Academy of Medicine (Singapore)* in 1999. The study evaluated the use of Minolest on lipid (fat) levels in people with high cholesterol and also evaluated its effect on obesity and blood pressure. Sixty-seven subjects received either Minolest (16.5 grams per day) or a placebo for 3 months. The individuals who took Minolest had a 3.24 percent decrease in their total cholesterol level and only a small (not significant) difference in the amount of weight lost or in triglyceride or blood pressure levels when compared with the placebo group. The subjects who took Minolest experienced few side effects and reportedly had reduced feelings of hunger and improved digestion.

COMMENTS: The three ingredients in Minolest have been shown to cause a feeling of fullness, reduce appetite, and result in some weight loss. See Part II for the entries for **psyllium, glucomannan,** and **guar gum** and how effective they are in assisting in weight-loss efforts.

FURTHER INFORMATION: **Print:** Tai, E. S., et al., A study to assess the effect of dietary supplementation with soluble fibre (Minolest) on lipid levels in normal subjects with hypercholesterolaemia. *American Academy of Medicine (Singapore)*, Mar. 1999, 28(2):209–13. **Web site:** Bionax at www.bionax.com.

More Than A Diet, by American Health

ACTION: Helps you maintain a lean body.
HOW SOLD: Tablets.
INGREDIENTS: Three tablets contain **chromium picolinate** and polynicotinate, 100 mcg; lipoactive factors (**L-carnitine, pyruvate,** inositol, choline, L-methionine, lecithin, phosphytidyl choline, phosphytidyl serine, taurine, betaine hydrochloride, vanadium vanadyl sulfate), 334 mg; amino-acid factors (**creatine monohydrate** L-lysine, L-glutamine, **L-phenylalanine,** L-tyrosine), 350 mg; herbal thermogenic factors (capsicum [**cayenne**], ginger, licorice, mustard seed, **green tea, American ginseng,** piper longum, **guggulpid,** suma, schizandra, astragalus, hawthorn, **kola nut, guarana,** 232 mg; fiber factors (oat bran, citrus punch, pulp cellulose, vegetable cellulose, beet fiber), 500 mg; herbal fluid factors (**uva ursi,** buchi leaf, couch grass, corn silk, hydrangea, juniper berries), 190 mg; essential fatty acids, 90 mg; appetite factors (citrimax [**garcinia cambogia**], **chitosan,** wheat oligio peptides, **gymnema sylvestre,** apple

cider vinegar, phaseoulus vulgaris), 550 mg; enzyme factors (coenzyme Q10, bromelain, lipase, protease, cellulose, aspergillus niger, aspergillus oryzae, FOS, pancreatin), 220 mg; fruit extract factors (apple, apricot, banana, cranberry, orange, lemon, lime, papaya, pineapple, strawberry, watermelon, grapeseed, grapefruit), 67.5 mg; vegetable extract (cabbage, celery, broccoli, brussel sprouts, yams, carrots, kale, collard greens, spinach, cauliflower), 50 mg. Contains no sugar, salt, starch, soy, dairy, artificial colors, flavors, or preservatives.

DOSAGE INFORMATION: The manufacturer suggests taking 1 tablet 3 times a day before each meal.

PRODUCT CLAIMS: The claims are that the dietary elements contained in this product are those needed to maintain a lean, healthy body. More Than A Diet "offers . . . what other dietary support systems have omitted."

COMMENTS: Although this product contains many ingredients that are known to supply nutritional benefits (for example, amino acids, fiber, and enzymes), the actual amount of most of them is unknown. Therefore, it is uncertain whether More Than A Diet provides any significant nutritional support for people who are on a reduced-calorie diet. The few "appetite factors" in this product have not been proven to help with weight loss. Consult your doctor before taking this product if you are pregnant or breast-feeding or taking any medications.

FURTHER INFORMATION: **Web site:** www.mothernature.com.

New Grapefruit Diet, by Irwin Naturals/ Omni Nutraceuticals

ACTION: Suppresses appetite.

HOW SOLD: Capsules.

INGREDIENTS: Vitamin B$_6$, 25 mg; iodine (**kelp**), 150 mcg; chromate (**chromium** polyniconate), 200 mcg; and 774 mg of a proprietary blend that includes soy lecithin; grapefruit powder extract (40:1); cider vinegar fruit; Bioperine™ piper nigrum extract (95 percent piperine) fruit.

DOSAGE INFORMATION: For best results, the manufacturer recommends taking 1 or 2 capsules up to 3 times a day with 8 ounces of water and drinking 8 glasses of water daily.

PRODUCT CLAIMS: The advertisements claim that the New Grapefruit Diet contains the ingredients that made the original Grapefruit Diet so successful and "formulated them into an amazingly effective new program." The program includes a diet and exercise plan, which is recommended for use along with the New Grapefruit Diet.

The claims are that chromium, lecithin, and Bioperine™ enhance the effectiveness of the product. Bioperine™ is a patented black pepper extract that is sometimes prescribed for flatulence, heartburn, and diarrhea. Lecithin helps disperse fats in the body's fluids and decreases the amount of saturated fat stored in the body. Chromium reduces cravings for sugars and other carbohydrates and helps metabolize sugars.

COMMENTS: There are no reliable scientific studies to support the claims made about this product. If you have diabetes and are taking insulin or any antidiabetic medications, consult with your physician before taking this or any product that contains chromium. Chromium has the ability to lower insulin resistance, alter the type or amount of medication needed to control diabetes, and change the frequency with which blood-sugar monitoring should be done.

FURTHER INFORMATION: **Web site:** See www.naturessecret.com.

NxTRIM, by Nova Pharmaceuticals

ACTION: Suppresses appetite and cravings for carbohydrates; also promotes urination.

HOW SOLD: Capsules.

INGREDIENTS: Two capsules contain the following ingredients: **L-phenylalanine**, 300 mg; St. John's wort, 50 mg; **ginseng**, 50 mg; L-glutamine, 50 mg; L-tyrosine, 100 mg; **L-carnitine**, 20 mg; **chromium** (chromate GTF), 100 mcg; niacin, 10 mg; vitamin B_1 (thiamine), 4 mg; vitamin B_2 (riboflavin), 4 mg; vitamin B_6, 4 mg; vitamin B_{12}, 166 mcg; calcium, 83 mg; magnesium 2 mg; zinc, 2 mg; bromelain, 25 mg; and **uva ursi**, 50 mg.

DOSAGE INFORMATION: The manufacturer suggests taking 2 capsules with water 3 times a day before meals.

PRODUCT CLAIMS: The manufacturer claims that "the all natural ingredients of NxTRIM form neuronutrients that work to restore brain chemical deficits." NxTRIM is described as a combination of amino acids, vitamins and minerals, herbs, and essential nutrients along with diuretics and digestive enzymes designed to help the body shed excess weight as well as replenish the body's essential amino acids and nutrients. It contains no artificial stimulants.

The actions of the primary ingredients are as follows: L-phenylalanine is a neurotransmitter that is claimed to reduce hunger and depression and increase memory and alertness. St. John's wort is an antidepressant that suppresses the appetite. Both L-glutamine and chromium reduce sugar and carbohydrate cravings, L-carnitine helps convert stored fat into energy, and L-tyrosine regulates the thyroid, which has an effect on metabolism and depression. Of the vitamins, B_1 aids in the digestion of carbohydrates, B_6 helps assimilate fats and proteins, and B_{12} plays a role in the proper utilization of proteins, fats, and carbohydrates. Uva ursi is the herbal diuretic that works without causing potassium loss.

The manufacturer conducted its own ninety-day double-blind clinical trial in which it compared NxTRIM (6 capsules per day) with a multivitamin-mineral supplement, which acted as the placebo. The study included forty-two overweight men and women. The researchers determined that NxTRIM "helped overweight individuals lose over 2.7 times the total amount of weight compared to a control group." The participants who took NxTRIM reported "an impressive increase in the amount of energy and stamina" and reduced hunger cravings. They were also twice as likely to successfully follow the diet plan prescribed by the researchers.

COMMENTS: The results of the study are questionable because it was conducted by the manufacturer and not by a nonbiased third party. In addition, several of the ingredients deserve comment. L-phenylalanine should only be taken while under supervision of a physician, especially at the relatively high doses in this product.

Individuals with the rare metabolic disorder phenylketonuria should avoid this product. The dosage of St. John's wort in NxTRIM is significantly lower than that usually considered to be effective.

If you have diabetes and are taking insulin or any antidiabetic medications, consult with your physician before taking this or any product that contains chromium. Chromium has the ability to lower insulin resistance, alter the type or amount of medication needed to control diabetes, and change the frequency with which blood-sugar monitoring should be done.

FURTHER INFORMATION: Web site:www.novapharmaceuticals.org.

ProVATE 1, by ProLab

ACTION: Stimulates metabolism.

HOW SOLD: Capsules.

INGREDIENTS: Three capsules contain: CreaVATE™, 1,500 mg (see explanation in Product Claims); sida cordifolia (6 percent **ephedra**), 416 mg; **guarana** extract (seed; 12 percent caffeine), 300 mg; white willow bark, 75 mg; **cayenne** (80,000 heat units), 75 mg. Other ingredients: magnesium stearate, gelatin, and microcrystalline cellulose.

DOSAGE INFORMATION: Package directions advise taking 3 capsules 2 to 3 times a day. The instructions also recommend not exceeding 3 capsules within a 4-hour period or 18 capsules within 24 hours, and not taking the capsules within 4 hours of bedtime as it may disturb the ability to sleep.

PRODUCT CLAIMS: The manufacturer calls ProVATE 1 a "technological breakthrough in the fight against fat." The Crea-VATE™ formulation is a high-energy molecule that bonds 60 percent creatine with 40 percent pyruvate, which reportedly provides superior metabolic efficiency. ProVATE also contains thermogenic agents, which help burn fat.

COMMENTS: This product contains **ephedra**, in the form of sida cordifolia, which has been linked with serious side effects, including death. It also contains a caffeine-containing substance, **guarana**. This combination is likely to cause anxiety, insomnia, agitation, and other reactions. See individual entries in Part II for details. In addition, there is no reliable scientific evidence that creatine and pyruvate cause weight loss.

Do not take ProVATE 1 if you are pregnant, breast-feeding, at risk of or being treated for high blood pressure; diabetes; pernicious anemia; nervousness; anxiety; depression; seizure disorders; stroke; prostate enlargement; or heart, liver, thyroid, or psychiatric disease. Avoid use if also taking an MAO inhibitor or any prescription medications.

FURTHER INFORMATION: **Web site:** See www.prolabnutrition.com.

Satietrol Natural Appetite Control, by PacificHealth Laboratories

ACTION: Controls appetite.

HOW SOLD: Powder in a packet (vanilla).

INGREDIENTS: One packet contains a proprietary formula of casein from whey protein; potato flour; sunflower oil; corn syrup solids; natural and artificial flavors; konjoc [**glucomannan**] flour; maltodextrin; **guar gum**; calcium lactate; sodium caseinate; soy lecithin; alfalfa powder; mono and diglycerides; dipotassium phosphate; sodium silicoaluminate; and aspartame. The nutritional breakdown is 80 calories, 30 calories from fat; 0.5 g saturated fat; 0 mg cholesterol; 6 g carbohydrates; 3.4 g fiber; 3.4 g protein; 120 mg calcium; 60 mg sodium; and 100 mg potassium.

DOSAGE INFORMATION:The package directions recommend mixing 1 packet with 6 to 8 ounces water and drinking it 10 to 15 minutes before each meal.

PRODUCT CLAIMS: This product claims to activate the body's appetite-control mechanism. The manufacturer explains that appetite is controlled by a protein called cholecystokinin, or CCK, which the body releases when you eat and which eventually makes you feel full. Satietrol has the ability to turn on CCK before a meal so you feel satisfied with less food and are less hungry between meals.

PacificHealth reports that three clinical studies have been done using Satietrol. In one double-blind, placebo-controlled study, Satietrol users were 35 percent less hungry 3.5 hours after eating than subjects who took a placebo. In a second study conducted over 4 weeks, subjects who took Satietrol reported a 32 percent decline in hunger 3.5 hours after eating. In a third study, researchers looked at the amount of weight lost over a 6-week period among subjects who took Satietrol. The average weight lost was 8.82 pounds, with some losing as much as 15 pounds. From this study, the researchers had evidence that the benefits of Satietrol use do not diminish with continued use. They also did not report any side effects associated with Satietrol use.

COMMENTS: Although the amount of each ingredient in this product is not revealed and the results of the studies may be biased, Satietrol may be a reasonably safe choice if you want to use it as a short-term diet aid along with a reduced-calorie eating plan and exercise. Both **glucomannan** and **guar gum** have demonstrated some effectiveness in weight loss, and the other ingredients in this product have not been shown to have adverse effects. Although no side effects have been associated with the use of Satietrol, it is recommended that you talk with your doctor before starting to take this product. Because this product contains aspartame, people with the metabolic disorder phenylketonuria should not use it.

FURTHER INFORMATION: **Web site:** See www.pacifichealthlabs. com and www.satietrol.com.

SeroThin, by Natural Balance

ACTION: Controls cravings.

HOW SOLD: Capsules (gelatin).

INGREDIENTS: Vitamin B$_6$, 7.5 mg; vitamin B$_5$ (pantothenic acid), 10 mg; **chromium**, 200 mcg (as DynaChrome™ Chromium, a trademarked chromium arginate/chelidamate); **L-phenylalanine**, 100 mg; tyrosine, 100 mg; St. John's wort, 50 mg; rhodiola, 50 mg; **citrus aurantium**, 20 mg; **5-HTP**, 15 mg. Inactive ingredients include gelatin, cellulose, and magnesium stearate.

DOSAGE INFORMATION: The manufacturer recommends taking 2 capsules 2 times daily with water, on an empty stomach.

PRODUCT CLAIMS: SeroThin reportedly reduces cravings and calms the nerves. Both the chromium and L-phenylalanine are claimed to reduce appetite, while chromium also helps reduce sugar and carbohydrate cravings. Citrus aurantium stimulates metabolism, 5-HTP produces early satiety, and St. John's wort has a calming effect.

COMMENTS: There is no reliable scientific research on this product that supports the claims of the manufacturer. The dosage of 5-HTP (60 mg daily) is less than the 150 to 300 mg or more shown to produce satiety, and the dosage of St. John's wort (150 mg) is far less than the 900 mg shown to improve anxiety and depression.

Before taking SeroThin, consult your doctor if you are pregnant, breast-feeding, taking MAO inhibitors or any prescription medications, or if you have any medical condition. This product is not for people younger than age eighteen. If you have diabetes and are taking insulin or any antidiabetic medications, consult with your physician before taking this or any product that contains chromium. Chromium has the ability to lower insulin resistance, alter the type or amount of medication needed to control diabetes, and change the frequency with which blood-sugar monitoring should be done. Individuals with the rare metabolic disorder phenylketonuria should avoid this product.

FURTHER INFORMATION: **Web site:** See www.naturalbalance.com.

---

7 Keto Naturalean, by Enzymatic Therapy

ACTION: Burns fat.

HOW SOLD: Capsules.

INGREDIENTS: One capsule contains iodine (potassium iodide), 100 mcg; copper gluconate, 500 mcg; manganese (Krebs cycle chelate), 500 mcg; 7 Keto **DHEA**, 100 mg; L-tyrosine, 100 mg; asparagus root extract (standardized 4.0 to 8.0 percent asparagosides), 100 mg; choline bitartrate, 50 mg; inositol (from rice), 50 mg. It does not contain any sugar, salt, yeast, wheat, corn, dairy, or artificial colors, flavors, or preservatives.

DOSAGE INFORMATION: According to the manufacturer, take 1 to 2 capsules per day with water.

PRODUCT CLAIMS: The literature claims that 7 Keto is an improved form of DHEA, which metabolizes fat, and that it is "clinically proven to burn fat and promote weight loss." The product also contains inositol and choline, which combine to form lecithin, another substance that metabolizes fat.

The manufacturer of 7 Keto Naturalean notes that their product was tested in a randomized, double-blind, placebo-controlled clinical trial conducted at Greenwich Hospital in Greenwich, Connecticut, by Carlon M. Cotker, M.D. Participants in the study who used 7 Keto along with a healthy diet and an exercise program lost an average of 1 pound per week compared with a placebo group, which lost less than ¼ pound per week. The results were attributed to increased levels of T3, a thyroid hormone that increases the basic metabolic rate. 7 Keto Naturalean consists of seven natural substances that support metabolism and thyroid function.

COMMENTS: This product contains **DHEA**, which is associated with significant side effects. In addition, the results of the study reported by the manufacturer are unimpressive, as 1 pound per week is the typical amount of weight lost when individuals follow a reduced-calorie diet and an exercise program, without the use of a diet aid.

FURTHER INFORMATION: **Web site:** See www.enzy.com.

SlimFast Weight Loss Shake

ACTION: Meal replacement.

HOW SOLD: Liquid shake, 11-ounce can. It comes in flavors: chocolate royale, dark chocolate fudge, fresh vanilla, milk chocolate, orange pineapple, strawberry & cream.

INGREDIENTS: The ingredients listed here are for the Chocolate Royale flavor; however, the content of the other flavors is very similar: skim milk; water; sugar; fructose; cocoa (processed with alkali); gum arabic; cellulose gel; calcium caseinate; vegetable oil (contains one or more of the following): canola oil or partially hydrogenated soybean oil); potassium phosphate; dextrose; soybean lecithin; cellulose gum; mono and diglycerides (emulsifier); carrageenan; modified cornstarch; artificial flavor; maltodextrin; vitamins and minerals; magnesium oxide; calcium phosphate; vitamin E acetate; niacinamide; sodium ascorbate; calcium pantothenate; zinc oxide; manganese sulfate; thiamine mononitrate; pyridoxide hydrochloride; vitamin A palmitate; riboflavin; folic acid; biotin; potassium iodide; sodium molybdate; chromium chloride; phylloquinone (vitamin K_1); sodium selenate; vitamin B_{12}; vitamin D_3.

The nutritional content is as follows: total fat, 3 g; saturated fat, 1 g; cholesterol, 5 mg; sodium, 220 mg; potassium, 530 mg; total carbohydrates, 38g (fiber, 5 g; sugars, 33 g); protein, 10g. All of the vitamins and minerals are present at 35 percent of Daily Value except for the following: vitamin K, 25 percent; folic acid, 30 percent; calcium, 40 percent; zinc, 15 percent; and selenium, 25 percent.

DOSAGE INFORMATION: The package instructions recommend replacing 1 or 2 meals each day with a shake, then eating sensibly the rest of the day.

PRODUCT CLAIMS: To stay slim, replace 1 meal per day, walk or exercise 30 minutes per day, and eat sensibly, including lots of vegetables and fruits. SlimFast is advertised as a balanced meal that includes 23 vitamins and minerals. Each shake contains 220 calories. The package notes that in place of a meal, many people use one can of SlimFast, a piece of fruit, and a noncaloric beverage.

COMMENTS: This product may help with weight loss and maintenance if it is used as directed. Do not use SlimFast as your sole source of nutrition.

If you are younger than eighteen, pregnant, breast-feeding, have health problems, or you want to lose more than 30 pounds, please consult your doctor before starting this or any other diet program. This product does not contain caffeine, preservatives, drugs, or chemical stimulants.

FURTHER INFORMATION: **Web site:** See www.slimfast.com for an interactive Web site.

Spirulina Herbal Diet Complex, by Rainbow Light

ACTION: Supports metabolism while dieting.

HOW SOLD: Tablets.

INGREDIENTS: One tablet contains **spirulina**, 200 mg; bee pollen, 10 mg; wheat grass, 75 mg; barley grass, 25 mg; **kelp**, 30 mg; echinacea, 40 mg; bayberry bark, 30 mg; nettle tops, 30 mg; cubeb berries, 30 mg; juniper berries, 30 mg; ginger, 30 mg; fennel seed, 30 mg; cleavers, 30 mg; **dandelion** leaf, 25 mg; hops, 25 mg; scullcap, 25 mg; butternut bark, 20 mg. Also contains 2:1 herbal extracts (92.5 mg) in a proprietary formula: burdock root; rhubarb root; **parsley** root; angelica root; sarsaparilla root; licorice root; dandelion root; **cascara sagrada** bark; vitamin B_6, 5 mg; **L-phenylalanine**, 25 mg; lecithin, 30 mg.

DOSAGE INFORMATION: According to package directions, take 1 to 2 tablets 30 minutes before or immediately after meals, or take 2 to 4 tablets in place of your midday meal.

PRODUCT CLAIMS: Spirulina Herbal Diet Complex, when used in conjunction with a weight-loss program, supports a healthy metabolism while you diet. It supplies non-fat green foods that satisfy the appetite; an herbal formula that assists with digestion and detoxifying; and nutrients for a balanced metabolism. The manufacturer recommends that you include many fibrous vegetables and grains in your diet when using this product.

COMMENTS: This product contains the potentially harmful substance **cascara sagrada** (see entry in Part II, pp. 48–50), although the exact amount is unknown. There is no reliable scientific research to support the manufacturer's claim that this product's formula supports a healthy metabolism or helps with digestion and detoxification. Individuals with the rare metabolic disorder phenylketonuria or who are allergic to bee pollen should avoid this product.

FURTHER INFORMATION: Web site: See www.rainbowlight.com.

Stimulife 750, by Stimulife International

ACTION: Suppresses appetite.

HOW SOLD: Caplets.

INGREDIENTS: Magnesium (magnesium oxide), 11 mg; zinc (zinc gluconate), 0.2 mg; selenium (selenomethionine), 0.06 mcg; **chromium picolinate**, 1 mcg; potassium citrate, 0.2 mg; and a proprietary blend (674 mg) consisting of: Dytrin (**citrus aurantium**); wheat grass (unjointed leaf); **guarana** extract (seed); damiana (leaf); goldenseal (leaf); gotu kola (aerial part); **ginseng** (root); cayenne pepper; fo-ti (root); ginkgo biloba (extract); hawthorn berry (fruit); white willow (bark); gingerroot; sarsaparilla (root); schizandra (berry); **uva ursi** (leaf); **green-tea** extract.

DOSAGE INFORMATION: The manufacturer recommends taking 1 to 2 caplets 45 to 60 minutes before meals and drinking 8 to 12 ounces of water. For individuals who weigh more than 200 pounds, a typical dosage is 3 caplets 3 times a day. The literature notes that "if what you are taking is not enough to curb the appetite or supply the energy you need, take more product."

PRODUCT CLAIMS: The wheat grass in the formula decreases appetite but does not kill it entirely. The formula also reportedly increases metabolism, enhances digestion, and provides nutrition-based energy (i.e., without the use of chemical stimulants). Two caplets contain the nutritional equivalent of 4 servings of fresh vegetables.

COMMENTS: There is no reliable scientific evidence to support the manufacturer's claims. Two of the ingredients in the proprietary formula— **guarana**, which contains caffeine, and **uva ursi**, which can cause liver damage—should be noted because the amount in the formula is unknown. If you have high blood pressure, diabetes, or are taking medication, consult your doctor before taking Stimulife 750. Do not take this product if you are pregnant or breast-feeding.

FURTHER INFORMATION: See www.stimulife.com.

Sunshine Slender, by Nature's Sunshine

ACTION: Meal replacement.

HOW SOLD: Powder, vanilla and cocoa-flavored, in a can.

INGREDIENTS: A proprietary blend of **medium-chain triglycerides; garcinia cambogia;** astragalus; ashwaganda; schizandra; reishi mushroom; proanthocyanidins (Grapine™, an antioxidant); soy; amaranth (a protein-rich grain). Each serving provides 190 calories; 28 g carbohydrates; 2 g fat; 15 g protein, and 6 g fiber (4 g soluble and 2 g insoluble). Also, vitamins A; E; B_1; B_2; niacin; B_6; B_{12}; pantothenic acid; C; D; biotin; folic acid; and the minerals calcium; magnesium; iron; copper; iodine; and zinc; plus phosphorus; manganese; selenium; vanadium; and potassium.

DOSAGE INFORMATION: The package directions are to mix 2 scoops (scoop provided) in 8 ounces water to make a balanced meal substitute; to use 1 packet for breakfast and another for lunch; and then to eat to a balanced dinner. Each product comes with a recommended menu plan.

PRODUCT CLAIMS: Sunshine Slender is a low-calorie meal substitute that contains medium-chain triglycerides, fats that, unlike other fats, are quickly absorbed and burned for energy. The presence of garcinia cambogia supposedly inhibits the storage of fat in the body by slowing down the conversion of carbohydrates to fat. The literature reports that this product was designed to help make meal planning easier for people who are dieting.

COMMENTS: There is no reliable scientific evidence to support the manufacturer's claims about the actions of the proprietary blend of medium-chain triglycerides and other ingredients. The product is dairy-free, low-fat, high-protein, and contains 35 percent of the Daily Value for all the vitamins and minerals listed except the last five.

FURTHER INFORMATION: **Web sites:** See www.healthy-sunshine. com and www.a-better-way.com.

Super Dieter's Tea, by Laci Le Beau

ACTION: Laxative.

HOW SOLD: Tea bags.

INGREDIENTS: Each bag contains **senna** leaves; orange peel; licorice root; althaea; **Siberian ginseng**; papaya; honeysuckle; chamomile; and spices. This product does not contain caffeine; sugar; yeast; artificial colors, flavors, or preservatives.

DOSAGE INFORMATION: The package directions advise pouring 16 ounces boiling water over 1 bag and allowing it to steep 2 minutes. A typical dose is 1 cup hot or cold after the evening meal; the second cup can be saved for the next evening. After 3 or 4 nights, the manufacturer suggests increasing the flavor by using 8 ounces boiling water per bag.

PRODUCT CLAIMS: This tea aids weight loss when used as directed.

COMMENTS: This tea contains **senna,** a powerful laxative that is recommended for relief of severe constipation, not weight loss. Whether this product contains an amount of senna that will cause side effects is uncertain. If you do decide to use this product, use it as directed: Do not drink more than 1 cup daily or use it if you have diarrhea, loose stools, or abdominal pain. Talk with your doctor if you are pregnant, breast-feeding, taking medication, or have a medical condition before you use this product.

FURTHER INFORMATION: See the information about "Dieter's Teas" in the introduction to this section. **Web site:** See www. natrol.com (maker of Laci Le Beau products).

Thermatol, by Matol Botanical International

ACTION: Burns fat, decreases appetite, increases energy.

HOW SOLD: Capsules.

INGREDIENTS: Each capsule contains a proprietary blend of bitter orange extract (**citrus aurantium,** Advantra Z™); ma huang (**ephedra**) extract; Citrin® extract (**garcinia cambogia**); **guarana** extract; **Siberian ginseng** extract; white willow extract; Atlantic

kelp extract; chromium chelate; inulin; bee pollen; octacosanol; alpha-lipoic acid; lecithin; **medium-chain triglycerides.**

DOSAGE INFORMATION: According to the manufacturer, take 1 capsule 3 times a day before meals.

PRODUCT CLAIMS: Matol claims that Thermatol's ingredients boost the body's ability to burn fat. Citrus aurantium supposedly helps burn fat; ma huang, white willow, kelp, and guarana boost metabolism; chromium helps reduce body fat; inulin helps prevent hunger; lecithin helps fat be dispersed in the body's fluids; medium-chain triglycerides suppress the appetite when the product is taken before meals; and octacosanol may increase your ability to exercise.

Thermatol is part of Matol's MBA™ Weight Management program, which also features meal-replacement bars and shakes and a product called Cell-Lean, which reportedly enhances metabolism and helps you sleep.

COMMENTS: This product contains **ephedra**, which has been linked with serious side effects, including death. It also contains a caffeine-containing substance, **guarana**. This combination is likely to cause anxiety, insomnia, agitation, and other adverse reactions. Generally, there is no reliable scientific research to support the claims made by the manufacturer.

If you have diabetes and are taking insulin or any antidiabetic medications, consult with your physician before taking this or any product that contains chromium. Chromium has the ability to lower insulin resistance, alter the type or amount of medication needed to control diabetes, and change the frequency with which blood-sugar monitoring should be done. Individuals who are allergic to bee pollen should note that this product contains an unknown amount.

FURTHER INFORMATION: **Web site:** See www.matol.com for information on Thermatol and other Matol weight-management products.

Thermo-Actives, by Natrol

ACTION: Boosts metabolism.

HOW SOLD: Capsules.

INGREDIENTS: Each capsule contains ginger extract, 150 mg; sida cordifolia, 100 mg; mucuna puriens extract, 100 mg; **cayenne**, 50 mg; mustard seed, 15 mg; Bioperine, 15 mg. Other ingredients include rice powder; silicon dioxide; gelatin; magnesium stearate: This product does not contain wheat; sugar; yeast; corn; soy; starch; artificial colors; or artificial preservatives.

DOSAGE INFORMATION: Package directions advise taking 1 capsule per day with a light meal.

PRODUCT CLAIMS: The advertisements claim that Thermo-Actives enhance the body's own natural metabolism levels. The formula contains various heat-producing herbs that generate a "spark" that burns calories without the use of chemical stimulants. Natrol's Thermo-Actives Plan includes the capsules plus a diet and exercise plan.

COMMENTS: One of the main ingredients in this product is sida cordifolia, which contains small amounts of ephedrine (**ephedra**). Ephedra has been linked with serious side effects, including death. Generally, there is no reliable scientific evidence to support the manufacturer's claims that the ingredients enhance natural metabolic activity.

FURTHER INFORMATION: **Web site:** See www.natrol.com.

Thermojetics Quick Start Weight Management Program, by Herbalife

ACTION: Meal-replacement program with nutritional and metabolic support.

HOW SOLD: The program consists of Formula 1 (French Vanilla, Dutch Chocolate, Wild Berry, and Tropical Fruit); Formula 2 tablets; Formula 3 capsules; TJ Green tablets; and TJ Beige tablets.

INGREDIENTS: Formula 1 protein drink is a specially formulated blend of soy proteins; vitamins; minerals; carbohydrates; and herbs. Formula 2 contains vitamin A and beta-carotene, 5,000 IU; vitamin B_1, 20 mg; B_2, 25 mg; B_6, 30 mg; niacinamide, 100 mg; B_{12}, 5 mcg; pantothenic acid, 20 mg; vitamin C, 150 mg; vitamin D, 400 IU; vitamin E, 30 IU; folacin, 400 mcg; biotin, 300 mcg; and more than 20 other nutrients. Formula 3 is a proprietary formula of potassium; magnesium aspartate; boron; silica; molybdenum; vanadium; gamma oryzanol; L-glutamine; chlorophyll; and pycnogenol. TJ Green tablets are a proprietary blend of **ephedra**, bladderwrack (**kelp**); yerba maté; valerian root; purple willow; fumitory herb; also papain and coating color FD&C Blue no. 1 Lake. TJ Beige tablets are a proprietary blend of hawthorn berry; **cascara sagrada; uva ursi**; alfalfa; corn silk; **parsley**; marshmallow root; magnolia bark; pau d'arco; pfaffia paniculata; astragalus; **fennel**; goldenrod; and licorice.

DOSAGE INFORMATION: The Herbalife Thermojetics Quick Start Weight Management Program is a comprehensive package designed to work together. According to the manufacturer, Formula 1, the Protein Drink, replaces 2 meals per day; Formula 2 suggests taking 1 tablet 3 times a day with meals; Formula 3, Cell Activator, is also taken 3 times a day—1 to 3 capsules with meals; and the TJ Green and TJ Beige are taken daily as needed to support the rest of the program.

PRODUCT CLAIMS: The literature claims the Protein Drink Mix provides 9 grams of protein per serving, all the essential amino acids, and helps you feel full so you won't crave unhealthy foods. It also contains "the breakthrough enzyme technology, Aminogen®, which acts to improve assimilation of dietary protein."

Formula 2 is billed as Herbalife's maximum formula multivitamin-mineral and herbal supplement that can help replenish a body that is faced with the assaults of poor eating habits, environmental toxins, and stress. The 39 vitamins, minerals, and Chinese herbs work together to "create a foundation for long-term good health."

Formula 3 is designed to boost the absorption of the vitamins and minerals you get from your diet. It also contains special trace elements that are involved in the Krebs cycle—a complicated series of enzyme-catalyzed reactions in the body's cells that involve the oxidation of carbohydrates, proteins, and fats.

The TJ Green and Beige tablets were designed to help "produce a desirable energy balance so excess body fat may be reduced."

COMMENTS: This weight-management program relies heavily on shakes and tablets and does *not* promote healthy, lifelong eating habits. The program is designed for quick weight loss, but maintaining the loss often proves difficult once people stop the program. Therefore, although most people do lose weight while on the plan, they usually regain it once they stop.

The TJ Green and Beige Tablets contain an undisclosed amount of **ephedra**, which has been linked with serious side effects, including death. They also contain unknown amounts of **cascara sagrada** and **uva ursi**, both of which can cause serious complications, and neither one of which is effective for weight loss.

FURTHER INFORMATION: **Web site:** See www.herbalife.com.

ThermoSlim 2000, by DRS & Co.

ACTION: Burns fat, suppresses appetite, boosts energy.

HOW SOLD: Six-hour time-release capsules.

INGREDIENTS: White willow bark, 50 mg; **chromium picolinate,** 200 mcg; **garcinia cambogia,** 100 mg; **guarana,** 250 mg; sida cordifolia, 100 mg; **ephedra,** 334 mg.

DOSAGE INFORMATION: A typical dosage is 1 capsule in the morning and 1 in midafternoon with water. The instructions recommend not exceeding 4 capsules within a 24-hour period.

PRODUCT CLAIMS: The metabolism boosters are white willow, guarana, sida cordifolia, and ephedra, while chromium reduces carbohydrate cravings and **garcinia cambogia** controls appetite. The advertisements claim you "can lose as much as 3 to 5 pounds per week" and that you "will see and feel immediate results the first day." Another claim is that "seven out of ten people prefer Thermo Slim 2000 instead of Metabolife," but no proof is given for this statement. Thermo Slim 2000 reportedly has no side effects and is "medically proven safe."

Another form of the product, X-Treme Thermo Slim 2000, is also available. It is advertised as being a "fiercely powerful blend of herbal ingredients and is therefore only recommended for sophisticated consumers." It contains the highest allowable percentage of ephedra and sida cordifolia, an herb that also contains ephedrine.

COMMENTS: This product contains a very high amount of **ephedra**, which has been linked with serious side effects, including death; and a lesser but significant amount of sida cordifolia, which contains ephedrine. Another ingredient in this product is the caffeine-containing substance **guarana**. This combination is likely to cause anxiety, insomnia, agitation, and other adverse reactions.

This product is not intended for people younger than eighteen years of age. Do not take it if you are pregnant or breastfeeding; if you are taking medication for high blood pressure; if you have heart or thyroid problems; or if you are taking MAO inhibitors or other prescription medications. While taking ThermoSlim, reduce or eliminate your intake of caffeine products.

If you have diabetes and are taking insulin or any antidiabetic medications, consult with your physician before taking this or any product that contains chromium. Chromium has the ability to lower insulin resistance, alter the type or amount of medication needed to control diabetes, and change the frequency with which blood-sugar monitoring should be done.

FURTHER INFORMATION: **Web site:** Both www.exrun.com/tslim. html.

T-Lite Weight Loss with Energy, by TEW Nutraceuticals

ACTION: Stimulates metabolism.
HOW SOLD: Capsules.
INGREDIENTS: Chromium chelate, 60 mcg; **chromium picolinate,** 60 mcg; vitamin B$_{12}$, 200 mcg. The proprietary blend includes **kola nut** concentrate (80 mg natural caffeine); potassium citrate; bladderwrack [**kelp**] algae; **Siberian ginseng**; wintergreen

leaf; gingerroot; gotu kola; ginkgo biloba; hawthorn berry; capsicum (**cayenne**); **cascara sagrada bark**; and **kelp** powder.

DOSAGE INFORMATION: According to the manufacturer, take 1 to 2 capsules 3 times a day with water before each meal. The instructions recommend not taking T-Lite past 4 P.M. as it may make falling asleep difficult, and not taking more than 8 capsules per day.

PRODUCT CLAIMS: T-Lite is advertised as a product that works with any diet program, but the manufacturer recommends their 3-day diet program, which they provide with the product. The combination of foods listed in the T-Lite diet program reportedly breaks down fat. T-Lite claims you can "lose up to 10 pounds in three days or your money back."

COMMENTS: This product contains **cascara sagrada**, which is a potent laxative that should be used only for severe constipation. See entry in Part II, pp. 48–50, for details.

If you have diabetes and are taking insulin or any antidiabetic medications, consult with your physician before taking this or any product that contains chromium. Chromium has the ability to lower insulin resistance, alter the type or amount of medication needed to control diabetes, and change the frequency with which blood-sugar monitoring should be done.

If you have high blood pressure; heart or thyroid disease; diabetes; prostate enlargement; or are taking MAO inhibitors or any prescription medication, consult your doctor before taking T-Lite. Stop taking T-Lite if you experience tremors, loss of appetite, nausea, sleeplessness, or nervousness. Because this product contains cascara sagrada, do not use it if you have diarrhea, colitis, loose stools, or abdominal pain.

FURTHER INFORMATION: **Web site:** www.drugstore.com/products.

Tonalin CLA 750 mg, by Natrol

ACTION: Reduces body fat.
HOW SOLD: Softgels.
INGREDIENTS: One softgel contains Tonalin® (60 to 70 percent **CLA**), 750 mg; **chromium picolinate**, 75 mcg; capsicum

(**cayenne**), 100 mcg; gingerroot, 100 mg. Other ingredients include beeswax; soybean oil; gelatin; and lecithin. This product does not contain eggs or glutens.

DOSAGE INFORMATION: The package directions suggest taking 1 to 4 softgels daily, preferably with low-or nonfat milk for maximum protein absorption. Protein-fortified soymilk also can be used.

PRODUCT CLAIMS: Conjugated linoleic acid reportedly reduces body fat, chromium picolinate reduces cravings and helps reduce body fat, cayenne stimulates metabolism, and ginger aids digestion. Natrol claims that years of research conducted at the University of Wisconsin show that CLA may be instrumental in reducing body fat and increasing muscle tone. Natrol's Tonalin CLA is the only patented form of CLA.

COMMENTS: Despite Natrol's claims about CLA, the majority of studies have been done in animals; thus, reliable scientific evidence to support its claims are lacking. If you have diabetes and are taking insulin or any antidiabetic medications, consult with your physician before taking this or any product that contains chromium. Chromium has the ability to lower insulin resistance, alter the type or amount of medication needed to control diabetes, and change the frequency with which blood-sugar monitoring should be done.

FURTHER INFORMATION: **Web site:** See www.natrol.com.

TrimBoost, by Natural BodyLines

ACTION: Fat absorber, metabolic stimulant.

HOW SOLD: Tablets (homeopathic remedy).

INGREDIENTS: **Chitosan**, 250 mg; **chromium** polynicotinate, 200 mcg; country mallow extract (10 percent alkaloids), 120 mg; **green-tea** extract (20 percent naturally occurring caffeine), 200 mg; Panax **ginseng** extract (root; 4 percent ginsenosides), 250 mg; enzyme digestive blend (amylase, amyloglucosidase, cellulose, lipase, protease, acid protease), 100 mg. Other ingredients include dicalcium phosphate; microcrystalline cellulose; croscarmellose sodium; stearic acid; silica; magnesium stearate; pharmaceutical glaze.

DOSAGE INFORMATION: A typical dosage is 1 tablet 30 minutes before meals with water. The manufacturer also recommends following a sensible diet and exercise program.

PRODUCT CLAIMS: The literature claims that the green tea, ginseng, and mallow extracts work together to raise the basal metabolic rate and body temperature slightly, which results in extra calories being burned. "TrimBoost nutritionally supports your ability to get control of your desire to eat," which in turn makes it easier to eat a healthy diet. The literature also claims that a major challenge facing manufacturers of supplements is finding a way to incorporate digestive enzymes with other nutrients in a way that prevents the enzymes from breaking down other ingredients in the product. The manufacturers of TrimBoost claim they use an advanced tableting method called bilayer technology, which separates the herbal extracts and the chromium in one layer and the enzymes and chitosan fiber in another. The result, they say, is better potency throughout the product's shelf life.

COMMENTS: The main ingredient, **chitosan**, has been shown to have minimal to no effect on weight loss. If you have diabetes and are taking insulin or any antidiabetic medications, consult with your physician before taking this or any product that contains chromium. Chromium has the ability to lower insulin resistance, alter the type or amount of medication needed to control diabetes, and change the frequency with which bloodsugar monitoring should be done.

FURTHER INFORMATION: **Web site:** See www.naturalbodylines.com.

Trim-Maxx Tea, by Body Breakthrough

ACTION: Laxative.

HOW SOLD: Tea bags. Comes in several flavors, including lemon, cinnamon, ginseng, orange, cran-blueberry, and original.

INGREDIENTS: Locust plant [**senna**]; gynostemma; lycii berry leaf; other ingredients depend on the flavor purchased.

DOSAGE INFORMATION: The manufacturer suggests placing 1 tea bag into 3 to 4 cups boiling water and allowing it to steep for 2 to 3 minutes. A typical dosage is 1 cup before bedtime; the rest can be saved for subsequent evenings.

PRODUCT CLAIMS: The packaging has a reminder that this product can increase bowel movement during the first week of use and that this response to the tea is a cleansing action that eliminates excess toxins and unwanted gas pockets.

COMMENTS: The packaging lists "locust plant" in the ingredients, which is senna. Senna is a potent laxative that is used to treat severe constipation; it is not recommended for weight loss. Elsewhere on the package it does say that the tea contains senna, but if you do not know that locust plant and senna are two names for the same plant, this information is confusing. This product is an example of why it is important to read labels carefully.

FURTHER INFORMATION: See A Few Words About Dieter's Teas in the Introduction to Part III. **Web site**: This product is available through various Internet sources, including www. mothernature.com.

Trimtime Orange, by Alvita

ACTION: Stimulates metabolism.

HOW SOLD: Tea bags. Comes in flavors: orange, cinnamon spice, peppermint, lemon.

INGREDIENTS: **Green tea** and green-tea extract; natural lemon flavor; red date extract; **ephedra**; white willow bark; gingerroot; **cayenne** extract; ascorbic acid; orange peel extract; rose hip extract; lemon peel extract; cardamom extract; cinnamon extract; acerola.

DOSAGE INFORMATION: Package instructions advise placing 1 tea bag in no more than 6 ounces boiling water and allowing it to steep for 3 minutes. Add honey to sweeten if desired.

PRODUCT CLAIMS: The ephedra, green tea (caffeine), and cayenne help boost the metabolism. The manufacturer notes that this product provides the best results when it is used along with a calorie-restricted diet and exercise.

COMMENTS: This product contains an undisclosed amount of **ephedra,** which has been linked with serious side effects, including death. It also contains caffeine (green tea). This combination is likely to cause anxiety, insomnia, agitation, and other reactions.

FURTHER INFORMATION: See A Few Words About Dieter's Teas in the Introduction to Part III. **Web site:** See www.alvita.com.

TrimTone, by Natural Health Company

ACTION: Stimulates metabolism, suppresses appetite.

HOW SOLD: Capsules.

INGREDIENTS: TrimTone contains **5-HTP,** 50 mg; vitamin C, 30 mg; and vitamin B_6, 15 mg; and a proprietary blend (1,100 mg) that includes L-arginine; L-lysine; L-ornithine; and **L-carnitine.** There are no artificial colors, flavors, preservatives, or added fillers.

DOSAGE INFORMATION: A typical dosage is 2 to 4 capsules before bed with 8 ounces of water.

PRODUCT CLAIMS: The 5-HTP controls appetite and cravings; L-ornithine metabolizes fat when taken with arginine and carnitine; L-lysine reverses the development of fatty deposits; and L-carnitine prevents fatty buildup.

COMMENTS: There are several scientific studies that suggest **5-HTP** helps control appetite and cravings for carbohydrates. Because this product contains several amino acids, it is suggested that you ask your doctor whether you should also take a general amino-acid supplement while you take TrimTone.

FURTHER INFORMATION: **Web site:** www.naturalhealthco.com/weightloss.htm.

TwinFast, by TwinLab

ACTION: Meal replacement.

HOW SOLD: Powdered shake in vanilla, chocolate, and strawberry.

INGREDIENTS: Calcium caseinate; crystalline pure fructose; egg white protein; cocoa; potassium phosphate; **guar gum** fiber; calcium carbonate; sodium chloride; potassium chloride; magnesium oxide; potassium citrate; aspartame (Nutrasweet brand); choline bitartrate; zinc gluconate; inositol; ascorbic acid; ferrous fumarate; manganese gluconate; selenomethionine; vitamin E; succinate; niacinamide; copper gluconate; D-calcium pantothenate; vitamin A (acetate); cyanocobalamin; pyridoxine hydrochloride; riboflavin; thiamine mononitrate; chromium chloride; vitamin D_3; vitamin K; sodium molybdate; folic acid; D-biotin; potassium iodide. All nutrients are present at 35 percent of Daily Value except for the following: selenium, 50 mcg; manganese, 1.4 mg; chromium, 50 mcg; molybdenum, 60 mcg; chloride, 440 mg; choline, 34 mcg; inositol, 34 mg; and vitamin K, 34 mcg.

DOSAGE INFORMATION: To prepare the shake, the package directions advise adding 1 level scoop (the scoop is provided in the package) of powder to 8 ounces cold water and stirring well. For fast weight loss, the manufacturer suggests using TwinFast 2 times daily in place of breakfast and lunch and eating a nutritious, well-balanced dinner that totals 560 calories. This plan (2 meals replaced with TwinFast, one 560-calorie dinner, and no snacks) supplies 800 calories per day. To maintain weight loss, the directions advise using TwinFast daily in place of either breakfast or lunch and eating a nutritionally balanced diet for the other 2 meals. Regular exercise should accompany both plans.

PRODUCT CLAIMS: The shakes replace meals and so restrict the amount of calories you consume. If the weight-loss plan is followed as recommended, the total daily caloric intake is 800 calories.

COMMENTS: The extremely low-caloric intake recommended by the TwinFast plan (800 calories) is considered to be dangerously low by many experts. Therefore, if you do want to use this product, it should only be done under medical supervision. This product should never be used as the sole source of nutrition. Consult your doctor before starting this or any weight-reduction plan, especially if you have high blood pressure; pernicious anemia; diabetes; heart, liver, kidney, or thyroid disease; any other disease; or if you are pregnant, breast-feeding, younger than eighteen years of age, or are taking prescription medication.

When added to water, TwinFast is suitable for those who are lactose intolerant. Three servings daily provide 100 percent of the recommended amounts of protein, essential vitamins and minerals, trace elements, and electrolytes.

FURTHER INFORMATION: See **Web site:** www.twinlab.com.

Ultra D Formula, by Cytodyne

ACTION: Fat burner.

HOW SOLD: Capsules. The product comes in five forms: Trial (if you want to lose up to 7 pounds); Regular (up to 15 pounds); Super (up to 25 pounds); Intensive (up to 35 pounds); and Super Intensive (more than 40 pounds).

INGREDIENTS: Bromelin; mint leaves; parsley; pancreatine; protease; amylase; lipase; papalin. Contains no sugar; starch; yeast; artificial colors, flavors, or preservatives.

DOSAGE INFORMATION: According to the manufacturer, take 1 capsule with a large amount of water before two of your largest meals.

PRODUCT CLAIMS: The manufacturer claims that Ultra D capsules "trigger the fat-burning process and eliminate all the excess fat from your body." This process reportedly keeps working even if you continue to eat normally. The manufacturer claims Ultra D Formula is "guaranteed to make you lose 15 pounds in two weeks" without the need for strenuous exercise or workouts or severe dieting. This is reportedly achieved because the "lipohylized enzyme capsules trigger the fat-burning process and literally force a body to lose weight without effort and within a few days." After losing the first 15 pounds during the first 14 days, the product promises that you will lose up to 4 to 7 pounds every subsequent week.

Ads for Ultra D Formula say that European researchers (unnamed) discovered rare botanical enzymes that consist of a substance called flavoprotein. To be effective, these enzymes must be dissolved and concentrated through a process called lipohylization, which is the basis for the product. These enzymes reportedly dissolve and eliminate fat cells and then convert them into energy.

COMMENTS: The manufacturer makes unrealistic claims that have no reliable scientific evidence to support them.

FURTHER INFORMATION: **Web site:** See www.interdietcenter.com.

Weightless Tea, by Traditional Medicinals

ACTION: Diuretic

HOW SOLD: Tea bags; available in flavors, cranberry and original.

INGREDIENTS: **Fennel** seed; hibiscus flower; lemongrass; **uva ursi** leaf; lemon verbena leaf; flaxseed; spearmint leaf; cleavers herb; red clover top; **parsley** leaf; buchu leaf; and natural flavors.

DOSAGE INFORMATION: Package directions advise adding 1 tea bag to 8 ounces boiling water and allowing it to steep 3 to 5 minutes. A typical dosage is 1 to 2 cups per day.

PRODUCT CLAIMS: This tea is a blend based on a traditional European mixture used to support internal cleansing and dieting by stimulating the metabolism. The basis of the formula is the fennel and hibiscus combination, which increases the metabolism rate and kidney function and facilitates bowel and urinary secretion. The addition of the other herbs enhances these processes.

COMMENTS: The claims made by the manufacturer are largely based on long-held herbal traditions and anecdotal reports. It is likely that this product can be safely used as a diuretic if used as directed. The only questionable ingredient is uva ursi, which can cause liver problems if used in large doses. Regardless of the product's safety, however, is the fact that diuretics provide only temporary weight loss and so are not recommended as a dieting aid.

FURTHER INFORMATION: **Web site:** See www.traditionals.com.

Weight Loss Plus Green Tea, by Optio Health Products

ACTION: Stimulates metabolism.

HOW SOLD: Tea bags.

INGREDIENTS: **Green-tea** leaves; **gymnema sylvestre** powder; cinnamon; orange peel.

DOSAGE INFORMATION: According to manufacturer's directions, place 1 tea bag in 8 ounces boiling water and allow it to steep for 2 to 3 minutes.

PRODUCT CLAIMS: Green tea stimulates the metabolism.

COMMENTS: Recent scientific studies show that green tea boosts metabolism; thus this product, when used along with a reduced-calorie diet and exercise, may help with weight loss. Weight Loss Plus Green Tea contains a 50:1 green-tea extract from organically grown tea. This means it takes 50 kilos of dried leaves to yield 1 kilo of P60. P60 is standardized at 60 percent polyphenols, which are some of the beneficial substances found in green tea.

FURTHER INFORMATION: See A Few Words About Dieter's Teas in the Introduction to Part III. **Web site:** See www.gaines.com.

Weight-Less, by Future Formulations

ACTION: Assists fat conversion; supports adrenal and thyroid gland function.

HOW SOLD: Capsules.

INGREDIENTS: Weight-Less contains 500 mg **garcinia cambogia** (50 percent HCA) plus a proprietary blend of vitamin C; vitamin B_6; pantothenic acid; manganese; chromium GTF; **L-carnitine;** L-tyrosine; DL-phenylalanine; soy lecithin; **kelp; apple cider vinegar;** gingerroot, **cayenne;** fenugreek; and bioflavonoids.

DOSAGE INFORMATION: A typical dosage is 2 capsules with each meal, not to exceed 6 capsules per day. The manufacturer recommends using this product along with a sensible eating and exercise program.

PRODUCT CLAIMS: Weight-Less works on several levels to promote weight loss. It assists the body in converting fat into energy by supplying it with the nutrients it needs to burn fat rather than store it. It also supports the adrenal and thyroid glands, which play important roles in weight control. Both of these glands are responsible for where fat is stored on the body. Therefore, this product reportedly is "formulated to work synergistically to support the metabolic pathways that lead to weight loss" and to lose it in the "right" places.

Weight-Less is formulated to decrease the amount of fat the fat cells take in by converting fats and carbohydrates into energy instead of into fat. It also helps convert fat into fatty acids and to move these fatty acids into the mitochondria, the energy producers of the cells. Once inside the mitochondria, Weight-Less helps promote the burning of fatty acids into energy. The manufacturer notes that many users report having much improved energy levels when taking the product.

The creator of Weight-Less is James L. Wilson, N.D., Ph.D., who notes that although Weight-Less is designed to begin working immediately, you may not see weight loss for 1 to 2 weeks. However, some people do see a loss of inches before they lose weight. This product is "not a crash weight-loss capsule but a nutritional supplement formulated to support and enhance the body's natural ability to metabolize away fat."

COMMENTS: Research studies to support some of the claims made by the manufacturer are available on the Web site. However, the studies concern biological actions rather than the specific product and its effectiveness as a weight-loss product.

No side effects have been reported from use of the product. If you are taking any prescribed medications, consult with your doctor before taking Weight-Less. This product is not intended for individuals younger than age twelve. This product does not contain any artificial stimulants.

FURTHER INFORMATION: **Web site:** See www.futureformulations. com.

Weight-Less Triple Kit, by The Herbalist

ACTION: Supports body's efforts at weight loss by strengthening body systems.

HOW SOLD: Three different liquid extracts: New Choice, Renew-U, and Blubberwack.

INGREDIENTS: In New Choice: gotu kola, 1:2; ginkgo biloba, 1:1; **guarana**, dried seed, 1:5; **American ginseng**, fresh root, 1:2; **Siberian ginseng**, fresh dried root, 1:5; **kola** fresh dried nut, 1:5; sarsaparilla fresh dried root, 1:5; licorice fresh dried root, 1:5; cinnamon fresh dried bark, 1:5; **cayenne** fresh dried pepper, 1:10; fresh gingerroot, 1:2, all in a base of distilled water, grain alcohol (approximately 46 percent), and kosher glycerine.

In Renew-U: milk thistle fresh dried seed, 1:3; oregon grape fresh dried root, 1:2; **dandelion** fresh root, 1:2; dandelion fresh leaf and flower, 1:2; burdock fresh dried root, 1:5; echinacea fresh root, 1:2; yellow dock fresh dried root, 1:5; cleavers fresh dried herb, 1:5; wild indigo fresh dried root, 1:5; **fennel** fresh dried seed, 1:5; gingerroot fresh, 1:2, all in a base of distilled water and grain alcohol (approx. 50 percent).

The Blubberwrack formula contains bladderwrack fresh dried, 1:5; gotu kola fresh herb, 1:2; **kelp** fresh dried fronds, 1:5; licorice fresh dried root, 1:5; echinacea fresh root, 1:2, all in a base of distilled water, grain alcohol (approximately 45 percent), and kosher glycerine.

DOSAGE INFORMATION: Per the manufacturer, all three products are taken the same way: 30 drops in water 5 to 7 times daily until improvement is seen, then 30 drops in water 3 times daily.

PRODUCT CLAIMS: The Herbalist explains that the ingredients in New Choice increase energy and stamina; reduce stress; enhance brain function; and reduce cravings for carbohydrates, alcohol, tobacco, and caffeine. Renew-U is primarily a cleansing formula that enhances the body's ability to efficiently process and eliminate toxins and fats. It revitalizes the urinary tract, liver, and lymphatic system and strengthens and stimulates digestion. Its diuretic properties help eliminate excess water weight. The Blubberwack formula promotes a healthy metabolism and thyroid function. The herbs in this tonic boost metabolism, increase the ability to burn fat, strengthen the thyroid, adrenal, and pituitary glands, and improve the ability to cope with stress.

The Herbalist notes that excess weight places stress on the vital systems of the body, including the liver, kidneys, thyroid, and adrenals, making them weak and underactive and, in turn, making it difficult to lose weight. Weight-Less Triple Kit helps strengthen digestion, boost metabolism, lessen stress, and balance energy and sugar levels.

The Herbalist recommends that users of their product follow a healthy diet that includes at least 40 ounces of distilled or artesian water daily; fresh vegetable juices; whole grains; legumes; green leafy vegetables; sea vegetables; fish; fruits; nuts and seeds; and the addition of flaxseed and borage seed oils in the diet. Foods to limit or avoid include meats; caffeine; alcohol; salt; dairy; eggs; sugar; flour products and high gluten foods; and deep-fried foods.

COMMENTS: The dietary plan proposed by The Herbalist to be used by consumers of their products is an excellent example of what a weight-reduction/maintenance diet should be, which leads to the question: Does Triple Kit sufficiently enhance what can be accomplished by diet and exercise alone? There are no reliable scientific studies to support the claims made by The Herbalist. However, none of the extracts contain ingredients that are known to be unsafe when taken as directed, so consumers could try it to see if the product delivers on any of its promises.

FURTHER INFORMATION: **Web site:** See www.theherbalist.com.

Xenadrine RFA-1, by Cytodyne Technologies

ACTION: Stimulates metabolism, burns fat.

HOW SOLD: Caplets.

INGREDIENTS: Two caplets contain the following: **citrus aurantium** (standardized 4 percent synephrine), 125 mg; **ephedra** (standardized 6 percent ephedrine), 335 mg; **guarana** (standardized 22 percent caffeine), 910 mg; white willow bark (standardized 15 percent salicin), 105 mg; **L-carnitine**, 100 mg; L-tyrosine, 80 mg; gingerroot, 50 mg; and vitamin B5, 40 mg.

DOSAGE INFORMATION: A typical dosage is 2 caplets before breakfast and 2 at midafternoon, not to exceed 4 caplets per day. If you weigh less than 150 pounds, the manufacturer recommends taking ½ dose during the first week. Xenadrine should be used with a reduced calorie diet and an exercise program for weight-loss results.

PRODUCT CLAIMS: The manufacturer claims that "Xenadrine's advanced new thermogenic formula represents the most sophisticated natural weight-loss technology available. Its powerful thermogenic combination has been proven effective in numerous scientific studies."

Cytodyne Technologies notes that Xenadrine's formula has been clinically tested and proven effective in many scientific studies and that the results have been published in the *International Journal of Obesity*. The results of the studies indicate that Xenadrine's combination increases the rate of fat loss by up to 300 percent and that it is superior to most prescription weight-loss formulas by up to 29 percent. It also has been shown to prevent the regaining of body fat that is typically associated with a great deal of weight loss.

COMMENTS: This product contains **ephedra**, which has been linked with serious side effects, including death. It also contains the caffeine-containing substance **guarana**. This combination is likely to cause anxiety, insomnia, agitation, and other adverse reactions.

FURTHER INFORMATION: **Print:** *Intl J Obesity,* 1991; 15(5): 359–366; 1989; 13 (Suppl 1) (abstract 151); and 1994; 18:99–103. **Web site:** www.cytodyne.com.

Nutritional Supplementation

for Dieters

AMERICANS ARE chronic dieters, and the impact of dramatically reducing caloric intake, fasting, eating nutritionally deficient foods, and taking various drugs to help with weight loss can take a tremendous toll on the body, especially in terms of causing nutritional deficiencies.

The chronic use of laxatives and diuretics, for example, can cause you to lose a significant number of nutrients. Use of diuretics can lead to deficiencies of potassium (if you are not using nonpotassium-sparing forms), magnesium, and B complex vitamins. Laxative use can cause deficiencies of calcium, phosphorus, and vitamins A, D, E, and K. If you are consuming products that contain caffeine (and drinking tea, coffee, and colas as well), you are in danger of deficiencies of vitamin B_1 (thiamine), inositol, biotin, calcium, iron, potassium, zinc, vitamin E, vitamin C, and vitamin B_{12}. People who use Xenical (orlistat) are warned that this prescription weight-loss drug causes the body to lose fat-soluble vitamins, including vitamins A, D, E, and K, and so they need to supplement these nutrients when taking the drug.

Eating healthy, whole foods—lots of fruits and vegetables, whole grains, legumes, nuts, and seeds—should always be your first choice, whether you are dieting or not. Yet most people tend to grab what is quick and convenient, which unfortunately often includes foods that are less than nutritious.

Combine these possible situations and you can have the basis for a nutritional disaster. This is especially true of people who go on very-low-calorie diets (VLCDs) of 800 calories or less, which are deemed potentially dangerous by medical experts.

HIGH-POTENCY MULTIVITAMIN-MINERAL SUPPLEMENT

You can avoid nutritional deficiencies by taking a high-potency multivitamin-mineral supplement every day. An example of the ingredients found in a good supplement are shown in the accompanying table. If you are in good health and eat a reasonably nutritious diet, the recommended doses in the low end of the ranges for each nutrient should be sufficient for your needs. If, however, you fit into one or more of the categories explained in the section following the table, you should look for supplements that provide doses in the upper end of the ranges.

When shopping for multivitamin-mineral supplements, you will notice that some of them contain minute amounts of trace minerals—for example, silica, vanadium, and iodine. These are not necessary, so their absence or presence is not important to your overall health.

Some diet and weight-loss/management products contain adequate or superior amounts of nutrients that help maintain the body's nutritional integrity while you diet. If you are using one of these products (several examples are in this book), compare the nutritional information on the package with the foregoing table to determine which additional supplements you may need. Consult your physician, a nutritionist, or a professional who is knowledgeable about nutrition if you are uncertain about your nutritional needs and whether you are meeting them.

SPECIAL NUTRITIONAL NEEDS

Some people have special needs or situations that call for additional nutritional supplementation. If you fall into any of the categories explained in the following, you should consider

SUGGESTED HIGH-POTENCY SUPPLEMENT DOSES

NUTRIENT	RECOMMENDED RANGE
VITAMINS:	
Vitamin A	5,000 IU*
Beta-carotene (preferred over vitamin A)	5,000–25,000 IU
Vitamin B_1 (thiamine)	10–100 mg
Vitamin B_2 (riboflavin)	10–50 mg
Vitamin B_3 (niacin/niacinamide)	10–100/10–30 mg
Pantothenic acid (vitamin B_5)	25–100 mg
Vitamin B_6 (pyridoxine)	25–100 mg
Biotin (vitamin B_7)	100–300 mcg
Folic acid (vitamin B_9)	400 mcg
Vitamin B_{12}	400 mcg
Vitamin C	100–1,000 mg
Vitamin D	100–400 IU
Vitamin E (d-alpha tocopherol)	100–800 IU
Choline	10–100 mg
MINERALS:	
Calcium	250–1,500 mg[†]
Chromium	200–400 mcg
Copper	1–2 mg
Iron	15–30 mg[††]
Magnesium	250–500 mg
Manganese	10–15 mg
Molybdenum	10–25 mcg
Potassium	200–500 mg
Selenium	100–200 mcg
Zinc	15–45 mg

* Vitamin A comes in two forms: retinol and carotene. Beta-carotene is preferred because it is less toxic than retinol, helps decrease the risk of heart disease, and helps prevent certain cancers. Many multivitamin-mineral supplements contain both vitamin A (retinol) and beta-carotene. Women of childbearing age should limit their intake of vitamin A to 2,500 IU daily, as there is a risk of birth defects at higher amounts.
[†] Best to take as a separate supplement.
[††] Men and postmenopausal women typically do not need additional iron. They should choose a multiple supplement without iron.
SOURCES: *Encyclopedia of Natural Medicine, The PDR Family Guide to Nutrition and Health.*

supplements that provide doses in the upper end of the recommended ranges.

- Among aging individuals, the need for vitamin D increases as the skin loses some of its ability to produce this vitamin. With aging also comes a greater inability to fight off infection, which means antioxidant needs increase. Postmenopausal women have a greater need for calcium, and elderly men and women need additional vitamin B_6 and B_{12} to help their flagging digestive systems.
- Individuals who cannot digest milk products (lactose intolerance) or who have chosen to stop eating dairy products may need to take calcium supplements. Another alternative is to eat other calcium-rich foods, such as calcium-enriched orange juice, calcium-fortified soymilk and other soy products, and leafy greens.
- People who are on VLCDs usually need greater amounts of all vitamins and minerals, but especially calcium, iron, zinc, and vitamins E and B_6.
- Strict vegetarians and others who for religious reasons do not eat dairy products or eggs may need to take supplements of vitamin D and vitamin B_{12} along with calcium, unless they eat adequate amounts of leafy greens, soybean products, sea vegetables, and fortified grains, juices, and soymilk.
- Homebound individuals or people who live in nursing homes may need supplements of vitamin D because they are not exposed to the sun. This applies to people of any age who are in these circumstances.
- Some vegetarians who do not eat legumes may need to take additional zinc and iron because these nutrients are more readily absorbed from animal foods than from plants.
- People who smoke, who experience a lot of emotional or physical stress, or who exercise strenuously usually

need to take additional amounts of antioxidants, especially vitamin C.

- People who drink alcohol excessively are generally in need of additional B vitamins.

Your goal is to be healthy. If you choose a nutritious diet, an enjoyable exercise program, and prudently selected weight-loss aids, including a high-quality multivitamin-mineral, and combine them with positive emotional and social support, you will have the recipe for success.

GLOSSARY

Adrenal glands: Two glands located on top of the kidneys, which produce and release hormones such as adrenaline (epinephrine) and cortisol.

Alfalfa (*Medicago sativa*): A plant that is used as a nutritional supplement and a body cleanser. It is both a laxative and a diuretic, and provides fiber, protein, calcium, and beta-carotene.

Aloe (*Aloe barbadensis*): A tropical herb that is used to treat constipation and ease stomach disorders.

Alpha-lipoic acid: An essential cofactor (helper) in energy metabolism, especially the metabolism of glucose (sugar) and fatty acids.

Appetite suppressant: Any drug or natural substance that can be used as part of a weight-reduction program, which should also include exercise, a low-calorie diet, and behavior modification.

Ashwagandha (*Withania somnifera*): A small shrub grown in India whose leaves and roots are commonly used in Ayurvedic medicine and in other traditions to restore and strengthen the body.

Asparagus root (*Asparagus officinalis*): A member of the lily family, this herb is used as a diuretic and to encourage bowel movements. It also may cause sweating.

Astragalus (*Astragalus membranaceus*): Also known as the milk vetch plant, it contains polysaccharides that stimulate the immune system and strengthen the body by stimulating the metabolism.

Atractylodes (*Atractylodes macrocephala*): The rhizome of this herb is used as a diuretic.

Barberry (*Berberis vulgaris*): The root bark of barberry is used to treat constipation and aid digestion.

Bee pollen: This highly nutritious product of industrious bees is said to enhance energy and endurance, aid in weight loss, and relieve stress.

Beeswax: A natural product produced by bees and harvested from the honeycomb. It is often used in the preparation of herbal products, especially lotions and salves.

Betaine hydrochloride: Betaine is stomach acid and helps the digestive process.

Bioflavonoids: These compounds are found in the white pith of citrus fruits and other foods that contain vitamin C. They help boost the immune system.

Bioperine™: A patented black pepper extract that is used to increase the absorption of nutrients.

Bissy nuts: Another name for kola nuts.

Blood glucose: A sugar that is the main energy source for the body's cells. It is the primary sugar the body makes from the food you eat, especially carbohydrates.

Borage (*Borago officinalis*): An herb that grows wild in Europe. It is used as a diuretic and as a tonic for the adrenal glands.

Brindell berry: Another name for garcinia cambogia, which is also known as HCA, Citrin K, and CitriMax.

Bromelain: This protein-digesting enzyme is found in pineapple and helps improve digestion as well as reduce inflammation.

Buchu (*Barosma serratifolia*): This South African shrub contains an oil that is used as a diuretic.

Burdock (*Arctium lappa*): Burdock root is used to treat urinary-tract infections and skin disorders.

Chamomile (*Matricaria recutita*): There are three types of chamomile, but the German variety has been studied more than the others. It is used to relieve stomach disorders and relax the digestive tract.

Chlorella: This fresh-water green algae contains all the essential amino acids as well as fiber and many vitamins, minerals, and other nutrients.

Cholecystokinin: A hormone secreted into the blood by the upper small intestine, which then stimulates secretion of the pancreas. It plays a key role in controlling feelings of hunger.

Cholesterol: A fatlike (lipid) substance found in the blood, liver, muscle, and other tissues.

Cleavers (*Galium aparine*): The most common use for this herb is for stimulating and cleansing the immune system, especially when used in a tea.

Coleus forskohlii: An herb in the mint family that is used for treatment of asthma, menstrual cramps, and allergic conditions.

Corn silk: This natural diuretic helps maintain the health of the kidneys and small intestine and is effective in removing mucus from the urinary tract. It is beneficial for people who are on high-protein diets, because mucus is a side effect of such diets.

Couch grass: An herb, also known as dog's grass, whose rhizome is used as a diuretic.

Croscarmellose: This substance (technically a carboxymethylcellulose sodium) is commonly used in the production of supplementary tablets and capsules.

Cubeb berries (*Fructus cubebae*): An herb of Indonesian origins, it is used for indigestion.

Damiana (*Turnera diffusa*): Although perhaps best known as an aphrodisiac, the leaves of this herb are also believed to be a laxative and to help the digestive process.

Diuretic: Any substance, either pharmaceutical or natural, that increases the elimination of fluids from the body through urination. Because the loss of fluids also means a loss of essential minerals, such as sodium, potassium, calcium, and magnesium, it is important to replace these nutrients. Loss of potassium, in particular, can be detrimental to the heart; thus, it is best to use potassium-sparing diuretics when possible.

Echinacea (*Echinacea pallida*): The most common use for this herb is to fight bacterial and viral infections.

Ephedrine: A synthetically produced drug that is similar chemically to ephedra. Ephedrine is used to treat bronchial asthma.

Fenugreek (*Trigonella foenumgraecum*): A member of the legume family, which is useful in treating digestive disorders.

Flaxseed (*Linum usitatissimum*): This herb, also known as linseed, is used as a bulking laxative.

FOS (fructooligosaccharides): These naturally occurring sugars promote the growth of beneficial bacteria in the body.

Fo-Ti (*Polygonum multiflorum*): In traditional Chinese medicine, this herb (which is also known as polygonum and fleeceflower root) is often prescribed for a variety of ailments, including dizziness, insomnia, constipation, and sore back.

Ginger (*Zingiber officinale*): In addition to being a culinary seasoning, ginger is used for digestive disorders, motion sickness, and to relieve gas.

Gynostemma: This herb is used to strengthen the immune system.

Hawthorn (*Crataegus laevigata*): The flowers, leaves, and fruit of the hawthorn shrub enhance blood flow and is said to have a calming effect.

Horsetail (*Equisetum arvense*): This plant is rich in silica, which helps form collagen. It is often used for urinary-tract problems.

Hydrangea (*Hydrangea arborescens*): This flower's roots and rhizome are used as a diuretic. It is also known as seven barks.

Hypothalamus: The hunger and appetite control center of the brain.

Inulin: A fructose-based sweetener that is derived from the root of chicory. Inulin suppresses appetite and metabolizes slowly, which helps prevent hunger.

Iodine: A mineral that is essential for the health of the thyroid gland, which controls metabolism.

Juniper (*Juniperus communis*): Juniper berries are used as a diuretic.

Kava kava (*Piper methysticum*): A South Pacific pepper plant, whose roots and rhizomes are often used to make a beverage. Herbalists recommend it for its sedative properties, which do not appear to be addictive.

Krebs cycle: A very complicated series of enzyme reactions in the body that involve the oxidative metabolism of pyruvic acid, which is a key product in the metabolism of carbohydrates, fats, and amino acids, and in the release of energy. It is also sometimes called the citric acid cycle.

Lecithin: This essential natural compound is a main component of the cell membranes. It is composed of phosphorus, choline, and fatty acids. One of its many functions is to emulsify and transport fat.

Lemon balm (*Melissa officinalis*): An herb known for its antiviral, antihistamine, and antidepressant properties. It is used to treat depression, digestive disorders, tension, fever, and colds.

Licorice (*Glycyrrhiza glabra*): Licorice is widely used as a cough suppressant and to heal digestive disorders. Because it is very sweet, it is often used to mask the bitterness of herbal remedies.

Licorice root *(Glycyrrhiza uralensis)*: The root of this plant is used to treat digestive and stomach problems, as well as coughs, asthma, and sore throat.

Lipoactive factors: Substances that affect the lipids and include, among others, carnitine, pyruvate, lecithin, and vanadium.

L-lysine: An essential amino acid (must be obtained through the diet), which is found naturally in kidney beans, soybeans, split peas, corn, and potatoes.

Lipotropic agents: Drugs or other substances that act on fat metabolism by hastening the removal of or decrease of fat in the liver.

Magnesium stearate: An odorless, tasteless, inflammable white powdery solid used as a tablet lubricant in dietary supplements, an emulsifier in cosmetics, and a drier in paint.

Maltol: An antioxidant that affects the taste of foods and beverages. It has the aroma of fresh bread.

L-methionine: An essential amino acid that is involved in more than forty processes in the body.

Monoamine oxidase (MAO) inhibitors: A group of antidepressant drugs that appear to work by stopping the breakdown of neurotransmitters in the brain. MAO inhibitors generally have more and more serious side effects than other antidepressants.

Mustard seed (*Sinapis alba*): This herb enhances metabolism and supports weight-loss formulations to help thermogenesis.

Niacin: Also known as vitamin B_3, niacin is involved in more than fifty essential bodily processes, some of which include regulating blood-sugar levels and converting food into energy.

Nobiletin: A bioflavonoid found in citrus, especially oranges, and a component of citrus aurantium.

Octacosanol: A natural compound found in many plants, whole grains, and nuts. It comes from wheat germ oil and may increase the body's capacity for physical activity and endurance.

Papain (Papaya): A protein-digesting enzyme found in papaya. It may be useful in treating poor digestion, constipation, and food allergies.

Pau d'arco (*Tabebuia impetiginosa*): This extract from a tree by the same name is used as an antibacterial, antifungal, antiviral, and antiinflammatory agent.

Pectin: A fruit extract that is a source of fiber, which also has the ability to absorb liquids, and so is often used to treat diarrhea.

Pfaffia paniculata: Also known as suma, this herb is found primarily in the Amazon basin. It is used as a general tonic for many of the body's systems and as a calming agent.

Piper nigruin: The dried, unripe fruit of the plant is used as a culinary seasoning. It is prescribed for heartburn, flatulence, and diarrhea.

Polysaccharides: A group of complex carbohydrates that include starches and cellulose.

Precursor: Something that precedes something else.

Proprietary medicine: Any chemical, drug, or natural preparation used as a remedy for which the manufacturer or producer is protected against naming the composition or manufacturing process based on free competition.

Protease: An enzyme that splits proteins.

Pseudoephedrine: A synthetic decongestant drug similar to ephedrine, which is found in the ephedra herb. Pseudoephedrine is used to treat respiratory problems.

Pullulan: A little-known herb that enhances the effects of gymnema.

Rhodiola: A mild antidepressant; also has possible heart-protecting qualities.

Rhubarb: The root of this plant is used as a laxative. Although it is often included in weight-loss products, it also can stimulate the appetite.

Saponin: A form of carbohydrate that neutralizes enzymes in the intestines that may cause cancer. It boosts the immune system.

Sarsaparilla root: An herb that is used to treat urinary-tract infections and psoriasis. Sarsaparilla root promotes glandular balance, cleanses the urinary tract and colon, and as a diuretic helps with weight loss. It is also a popular soft-drink flavoring.

Schizandra berry: This member of the magnolia family has purple-red fruit that is used by Western herbalists to help the body deal with stress and to increase energy. Chinese medicine practitioners prescribe it for various conditions, including insomnia and skin problems. People who experience epileptic episodes or who are hypertensive should not take this herb.

Serotonin: A neurotransmitter found in the brain. It is involved in the control of appetite and moods. Low levels are associated with depression and overeating, whereas higher levels are associated with appetite control and better moods.

Set point: A weight the body tries to maintain despite one's attempt to lose weight.

Sida cordifolia: An Ayruvedic herb used to treat asthma and bronchial distress, edema, and headache. It contains ephedrine and pseudoephedrine, but in lesser quantities than is found in ma huang, so it is a weaker stimulant.

Skullcap or scullcap (*Scutellaria lateriflora*): The leaves and flowers of this plant are used for insomnia and to relieve nervous tension.

Slippery elm (*Ulmus fulva*): This herb is highly recommended for digestive disorders.

Stearic acid: A fatty acid that is extracted from tallow (beef fat) and used in the production of tablets and capsules.

St. John's wort (*Hypericum perforatum*): In addition to the treatment of mild depression, the flowers of this popular herb are used to boost the immune system.

Synephrine: A substance found in citrus, with the highest concentrations being in citrus aurantium and citrus unshiu. Synephrine is a decongestant and helps maintain blood-pressure levels. Although similar to ephedrine in that it can raise the metabolic rate and promote fat burning, it does not cause the agitation usually associated with ephedrine.

Thermogenic: Something with the ability to produce heat, especially in the body.

Triphala: This popular Ayurvedic herb is a laxative that cleanses and detoxifies without depleting the body's reserves.

L-tyrosine: This amino acid is a precursor of epinephrine, thyroxine (a hormone produced by the thyroid gland), and melanin. Tyrosine needs folic acid and ascorbic acid (vitamin C) for its metabolism.

Valerian root (*Valeriana officinalis*): An herb used for more than 1,000 years for its calming properties and as a sleep aid. Unlike

pharmaceutical sleeping aids, valerian does not cause morning grog-
giness and is not habit-forming.

Vanadium: Little is known about this trace mineral, although it
appears to help lower blood-sugar levels and to assist with cholesterol metabolism.

Wheat grass: A member of the cereal family, it is rich in vitamins,
minerals, chlorophyll, and trace elements.

White willow bark (*Salix alba*): This tree is a natural source of
salicin, which is used as a painkiller.

SUGGESTED READINGS

Balch, James F., and Phyllis Balch, *Prescription for Nutritional Healing*. Garden City Park, NY: Avery, 1993.

Brody, Jane, *The Good Food Book*. New York: Bantam, 1987.

Colbin, Annemarie, *Food and Healing*. New York: Ballantine, 1986.

Connor, William, and Sonja Connor, *The New American Diet*. New York: Fireside, 1989.

Cooper, Kenneth H., M.D., *Advanced Nutritional Therapies*. Nashville: Thomas Nelson, 1996.

Fraser, Laura, *Losing It: America's Obsession with Weight and the Industry that Feeds on It*. New York: Dutton, 1997.

Graedon, Joe, and Teresa Graedon, *The People's Pharmacy Guide to Home and Herbal Remedies*. New York: St. Martins, 1999.

Greenwood-Robinson, Maggie, *Natural Weight-Loss Miracles: 20 Wonder Pills, Powders and Supplements to Burn Fat and Shed Pounds Naturally*. New York: Penguin, 1999.

Grieve, Maud, *A Modern Herbal*. Volumes 1 and 2. New York: Dover, 1978.

Haas, Elson M., M.D., *The False Fat Diet: The Revolutionary 21-Day Program for Losing the Weight You Think Is Fat*. New York: Ballantine, 2000.

Larkin, Marilyn, "Ways to Win at Weight Loss." FDA Consumer #99–1287. Web site: www.fda.gov/fdac/reprints/weight.html.

Lappe, Frances M., *Diet for a Small Planet*. Rev. ed. New York: Ballantine, 1975.

Lu, Nan, and Ellen Schaplowsky, *Traditional Chinese Medicine: A Natural Guide to Weight Loss that Lasts*. New York: Avon, 2000.

McDougall, John A., M.D., *The McDougall Program for a Healthy Heart*. New York: Penguin, 1996.

———. *The New McDougall Cookbook*. New York: NAL, 1993.

———. *The McDougall Program: 12 Days to Dynamic Health*. New York: Penguin, 1991.

Mirkin, Gabe, M.D., *Fat Free, Flavor Full*. Boston: Little, Brown, 1995.

Mitchell, Deborah, *Natural Medicine for Weight Loss*. New York: Dell, 1998.

Murray, Michael T., N.D., *The Healing Power of Herbs*. 2d ed. Rocklin, CA: Prima, 1995.

———. *Natural Alternatives to Over-the-Counter and Prescription Drugs*. New York: William Morrow, 1994.

Nash, Joyce, and Linda Ormiston, *Taking Charge of Your Weight and Well-Being*. Palo Alto, California: Bull, 1978.

Ornish, Dean, MD, *Eat More, Weigh Less*. New York: HarperCollins, 1993.

Robbins, John. *Diet for a New America: How Your Food Choices Affect Your Health, Happiness, and the Future of Life on Earth*. Walpole, NH: Stillpoint, 1987.

Siegel, Bernie, M.D., *Peace, Love and Healing: Bodymind Communication and the Path to Self-Healing*. New York: Harper & Row, 1989.

Weil, Andrew, M.D., *Eating Well for Optimum Health*. New York: Knopf, 2000.

———. *Natural Health, Natural Medicine: 8 Weeks to Optimum Health*. Boston: Houghton Mifflin, 1990.

Werbach, Melvyn, M.D., *Healing with Food*. New York: HarperCollins, 1993.

———. *Healing Through Nutrition*. New York: HarperCollins, 1993.

Wilbert, Jeffrey R., and Norean K. Wilbert. *Fattitudes: Beat Self-Defeat and Win Your War with Weight*. New York: St. Martins, 2000.

Wurtman, Judith J., Ph.D., *The Serotonin Solution*. New York: Fawcett Columbine, 1996.

RESOURCE LIST

SUPPLIERS

There are hundreds of suppliers of diet and weight-loss products, including manufacturers, multilevel marketing companies, and distributors who often handle dozens of brands. The suppliers listed in the following are in addition to those listed in Parts II and III of this book and include distribution sites where you can often get discount prices.

Fresh Vitamins: www.freshvitamins.com
Swanson Health Products: www.swansonvitamins.com
EShop: www.eShopconnections.com
Planet Rx: www.planetrx.com
Mother Nature: www.mothernature.com
Discount Boulevard: www.discountblvd.com

GENERAL INFORMATION ON WEIGHT LOSS AND WEIGHT-LOSS FRAUD

Centers for Disease Control: www.cdc.gov/health/obesity.htm
Barbara's Obesity Medications & Research News (newsletter and Web site for professionals and consumers): www.obesity-news.com
American Obesity Association (research information): www.obesity.org

Best of Weight Loss (a directory maintained by specialists in weight loss, weight management, exercise, and Internet research): www.BestofWeighloss.com

Food and Drug Administration. Consumer advice on weight loss and nutrition: http://vm.cfsan.fda.gov

Weight-Loss Zone (offers free weight-loss resources): www.FreeWeightloss.com

Weight Directory (single point of navigation to the products and services you want to buy that can help you lose weight): www.weightdirectory.com

For information about weight-loss scams, see the following Web sites:

www.nutramed.com/weight/scams.htm
www.nutramed.com/weight/weightloss.htm
www.dietfraud.com
www.healthyweight.org/identify.htm
www.healthyweight.net
www.thriveonline.com/weight/diets/cautions.html

If you have a complaint about a nonprescription product or you believe the manufacturer is making fraudulent claims, you can contact the following organizations:

The Federal Trade Commission, which has jurisdiction over advertising and marketing of foods, nonprescription drugs, medical devices, and health-care services. The FTC can seek federal court injunctions to stop fraudulent advertising and obtain redress for consumers. Contact: FTC, Correspondence Branch, Washington, DC 20580.

The Food and Drug Administration (FDA) has jurisdiction over the content and labeling of foods, drugs, and medical devices. The FDA can take legal action to seize and stop the sale of products that are falsely labeled. Contact: FDA, Consumer Affairs and Information, 5600 Fishers Lane, Rockville, MD 20857.

Your **state attorney general** has the authority to investigate and prosecute unfair or deceptive acts and practices. Some, depending on the individual state's consumer protection statutes, also have the power to seek consumer restitution, civil fines, and revocation of a company's authority to do business. Contact: your State Attorney General, Office of Consumer Protection.

INDEX

Mucilage, 98
Mucus, 185
Mukul tree, 84
Multivitamin-mineral supplement,
    high-potency, 178, 179
Mustard seed, 187

NaturalMax Diet Plan, 137
Natural supplements,
    misconceptions about, 15
New Choice, 174
New Grapefruit Diet, 146–147
Niacin, 134, 179, 187
Niacinamide, 179
Nobiletin, 59, 187
Nursing homes, 180
Nutritional deficiencies, 6
Nutritional needs, special, 178,
    180–181
Nutritional product labels, reading,
    18–20
Nutritional supplementation for
    dieters, 177–181
NutritionBoost vitamins, 125
Nuts, 177
NxTRIM, 147–149

Obalan, 37–39
Obe-Nix, 35–37
Obephen, 35–37
Obermine, 35–37
Obesity, ix–x
    causes of, 6–8
    overweight versus, 2
Obestin-30, 35–37
Octacosanol, 187
Omega-6, 93–94
Ona-Mast, 35–37
Optimal Collagen Profile, 116
Orlistat, 33–35, 177
Over-the-counter single-ingredient
    weight-management products,
    43–104
    best bets, 45–46
    choosing, 44–45
    prescription weight-loss drugs
        versus, 43
Overweight, ix–x
    causes of, 6–8
    obesity versus, 2

P60, 172
Panax quinquefolius, 76–77
Panoxosides, 76
Pantothenic acid, 179
Papain, 187
Papaya, 187
Parmine, 35–37
Parsley, 95
Pau d'arco, 188
Paullinia cupana, 82–84
Pectin, 114, 188
Pennywort, 113
Pepper, 50
Permanent weight loss, xii
Pfaffia paniculata, 188
Phendimetrazine (phendimetrazine
    tartrate), 37–39
Phentermine (phentermine
    hydrochloride), 17, 35–37
Phentrol, 35–37
Phenylalanine, 96–97
Phenylketonuria, 151
Phenylpropanolamine (PPA), 96,
    97
Phenzine, 37–39
Phoenix-tail fern, 122
Phosphorus, 177
Physical examination, 9
Physical stress, 180
Physicians, v
Picolinic acid, 56
Pima Indians, 7
Piper methysticum, 186
Piper nigruin, 188
Placebo effect, 15
Plantain, 122
PM-300, 114–115
Point of Change (SM) weight-
    management program, 41
Polygonum, 186
Polygonum multiflorum,
    185–186
Polyphenols, 79–80
Polysaccharides, 188
Pondimin, 13, 17–18
Postmenopausal women, 179, 180
Potassium, 177, 179
Potassium-sparing diuretics, 185
PPA (phenylpropanolamine), 96,
    97

ABOUT THE AUTHORS

Deborah R. Mitchell is a medical writer and journalist whose articles have appeared in professional journals as well as national consumer magazines. She has authored or coauthored fifteen books about various health topics, including *The Natural Health Guide to Headache Relief*, coauthored with Paula Maas, M.D.; *The SAM-e Solution; MSM: The Natural Pain Relief Remedy; Natural Painkillers;* and *The Dictionary of Natural Healing*. Ms. Mitchell is an experienced collaborator, a meticulous researcher, and highly skilled at making complex technical information easy to understand. She lives and works in Tucson, Arizona.

David Charles Dodson, M.D., is Assistant Clinical Professor of Medicine at Tufts University School of Medicine. He specializes in clinical nutrition and the treatment of obesity and maintains a private practice based at the Newton-Wellesley Hospital.